Clinical Biostatistics

An Introduction to Evidence-Based Medicine

Graham Dunn and Brian Everitt

Institute of Psychiatry
London, UK

Edward Arnold
A member of the Hodder Headline Group
LONDON   SYDNEY   AUCKLAND

Copublished in the Americas by Halsted Press
an imprint of John Wiley & Sons Inc.
New York – Toronto

First published in Great Britain 1995 by
Edward Arnold, a division of Hodder Headline PLC,
338 Euston Road, London NW1 3BH

Copublished in the Americas by Halsted Press,
an imprint of John Wiley & Sons Inc.,
605 Third Avenue, New York, NY 10158

British Library Cataloguing in Publication Data
A catalogue record for this book is available from the British Library

ISBN 0 340 59531 0

1 2 3 4 5 95 96 97 98 99

Typeset by Wearset, Boldon, Tyne and Wear
Printed and bound in Great Britain by J. W. Arrowsmith Ltd, Bristol

Contents

Preface

As an increasing number of medical schools move over to a problem-based curriculum, in which clinical skills and basic science are learnt in an integrated manner, there is clearly a need for a biostatistics text which is also motivated by clinical problems. The present book has been written in response to this need. In the traditional medical curriculum great stress has been placed on the acquisition of knowledge and, to some extent, skills. Little attention is paid to the students' attitudes. This text, however, concentrates much more on influencing students' attitudes towards the use of evidence and, in particular, the appropriate and valid use of statistical inference in clinical medicine. Students will also acquire skills that are useful for the analysis of their own data (in student projects, for example) and, specially, for the clinical appraisal of the work of others. Little attention is paid to the mere learning of statistical formulae and other recipes. When we say in the text that the technical details (formulae, etc.) need not concern the student, we mean it. We are not being patronizing! We are much more concerned in influencing the way students think about the use of evidence than in teaching them how to manipulate impenetrable formulae. With the widespread use of statistical packages on personal computers much of the detailed technical knowledge and skill which may have been useful in the past is, in any case, no longer needed. We do not, however, provide any details of statistical packages as this information very quickly becomes out-of-date and quite misleading.

Although we hope that this book will be used as the main text for courses on the critical appraisal of statistical evidence in medicine, we also hope that it will stimulate students to look further afield for others' views on this subject; that the book will be the start of the student's questioning rather than the final word. Accordingly, we have provided recommended reading lists at the end of each chapter. A brief glance at this material will quickly reveal the important influence of David Sackett, Gordan Guyatt and their colleagues at McMaster University. Their work on problem-based learning and the teaching of critical appraisal, together with their advocacy of 'evidence-based medicine' has provided an inspiration for much of the present book.

One of the consequences of pursuing a problem-orientated approach is that statistical procedures that are routinely part of a traditional medical statistics syllabus have all but disappeared. Others have been given much greater prominence. One area that, perhaps surprisingly, we have chosen not to discuss in any detail, for example, is significance testing. This was not, at first, a deliberate decision, but it soon became obvious to us that significance tests simply did not provide the ideal solutions to the problems which we posed. We decided to concentrate on estimation and the construction of confidence intervals instead. We do eventually introduce significance tests in a Postscript, however, more because readers might be expecting to see them than because we have had second thoughts. An area which we chose to discuss in considerable detail, at least in comparison to the coverage in most existing texts, is that on assessing the quality of measurements. Additionally, we emphasize the importance of good design.

The text, we hope, could be read with profit by 'students' at all stages of their clinical careers. We make no assumptions about either any prior statistical knowledge or expertise in medicine. We have deliberately kept the technical discussion of any clinical problems at a level that could easily be understood by the lay person. In fact, we hope that non-clinicians (even patients or other users of health services) would find the contents interesting reading!

Finally, G.D. would like to thank Charles Engel and Roy Cox (Centre for Higher Educational Studies, Insitute of Education) for many stimulating discussions on the nature of teaching and learning in medical education.

Graham Dunn
Brian Everitt

May 1994

Clinical Problems and Statistical Solutions

1

1.1 INTRODUCTION

'To understand God's thoughts we must study statistics, for those are the measure of his purpose.'

Florence Nightingale (1820–1910)

Florence Nightingale clearly had a high regard for the subject of statistics and she may even have had similar views of statisticians. In today's more secular society this view might not be expressed exactly in this form, but the message would still be clear: statistics has a vital role in the understanding of our world. But nowadays not everyone is so convinced by this! On the ladder of the general public's affection, the professional statistician probably occupies a lowly rung close to traffic wardens and tax collectors. The subject of statistics itself is seen by the vast majority of people as dull, devious and even downright dangerous, whilst its practitioners are often classed as professionally unreliable and socially undesirable. Statisticians learn at an early stage of their career never to admit to other guests at parties just what they do for a living, otherwise they are as likely to find themselves as ostracized as accountants!

But in this text we hope to convince you that statistics is both useful and interesting. By presenting you with a series of simple clinically important questions or problems, and by showing you how these questions might be answered through the use of statistical methods, we aim to demonstrate the fundamental importance of statistical thinking in modern medicine. This applies, not just in medical research, but also in routine clinical practice and decision-making with regard to health service provision and more general problems of public health. In reading this book and working through the exercises, we hope you will also pick up a few statistical skills and knowledge of the use and interpretation of statistical methods. Our primary aim is that you learn to understand what statistical methods are for, and begin to learn the vocabulary and grammar of a language in which you can question empirical statements concerning the nature of the clinical world. Consequently technical details of the methods are mostly confined to the Displays; in the body of the text such details are kept to their essential minimum.

1.2 EVIDENCE, STATISTICS AND THE SCIENTIFIC METHOD

The distinguishing feature of modern science is *scepticism*: we are no longer prepared to take the pronouncements of authority on trust. We ask for evidence and we wish to evaluate the claims of experts (whether they be scientists, clinicians or politicians) in light of this evidence. If an eminent molecular biologist claims that vitamin C cures the common cold then we wish to test his claims through experiment. We *may* be inclined to take his views seriously because of his scientific reputation, but we test his views by observation of the effects of vitamin C on patients, rather than simply accepting his authority without question. A similar approach should be taken in the evaluation of all possible therapies, whether they be high-tech surgical procedures, herbal remedies, or psychotherapies. In particular, they should not be assumed to be beneficial just because they are new! This healthy scepticism should also influence our views concerning the nature and cause of illnesses, on the one hand, and to approaches to reform the administration of health service provision, on the other. In all situations we should be demanding to see the evidence that a particular claim is merited so that we can assess its validity for ourselves.

The scientific approach to medicine demands that we question claims about health and illness by recourse to observation and experiment. We check claims against the empirical evidence. In order to be able to do this, we need to be able to understand the nature of the evidence (*the data*) and the way in which it has been collected and presented. We do not necessarily need to carry out research ourselves, but we must be able to understand and evaluate the outcome of that research. This does not mean, however, that we will be in a position to challenge the work of clinical scientists, but we will be able to understand the reasoning behind their work, be aware of possible methodological traps, and decide for ourselves how much trust to put in their findings. We will also be able to follow the arguments and criticisms produced by others.

Statistics is one of the core components of modern scientific method. It is the discipline primarily concerned with the logic of the design of experiments and surveys. It is also the subject concerned with the methodology of data presentation and with the use of the data in decision making and scientific inference. It is inevitably mathematical, but the level of mathematics need not be highly technical or sophisticated. In the hands of an honest scientist or clinician there is nothing suspect or devious about the use of statistical methods. The aim here is to use statistical thinking to get at the truth, not to hide it or otherwise to deceive a third party. Statistical methods *can*, however, be used in devious ways to bolster defective arguments or to sell apparently useless products. This is not a problem for statistics, as such, but for the unsuspecting reader. The user of statistics can also make mistakes—he or she may not have fully understood the way in which a particular statistical method should or should not have been used. There need not have been any devious intent. Whether or not you suspect the abuse of statistics, always question the way in which the evidence has been collected and presented. Never accept anything at face value. Ask the following questions:

- Are the claims backed by empirical evidence or just the supposed authority of the author?
- How has this evidence been collected? Is it merely anecdotal or have data been collected systematically? If an experiment or survey has been used, how was it conducted? Are there faults in the design? Are the patients representative? Is there something atypical about the setting of the research?
- How have the data been summarized and presented? Is it appropriate to present the data in this way?
- How are the data used to support the author's claims? Are the statistical arguments valid or flawed?
- Are there other, perhaps more convincing, explanations for the results? Has the author seriously considered and discounted the alternatives?

1.3 STATISTICS IN THE MEDICAL LITERATURE

Most clinicians in the United Kingdom, and many in the rest of the world, read either the *British Medical Journal* (BMJ) or the *Lancet*. In the United States of America the equivalent might be the *Journal of the American Medical Association* (JAMA) or the *New England Journal of Medicine*. Nowadays journals and magazines for clinicians are increasingly filled with statistical topics, since statistics are increasingly a part of medical practice. No doctor can escape the demands of audit, resource allocation, hospital utility, vaccination uptake and the like. The reader of the BMJ, the *Lancet* and similar journals will find themselves bombarded with vital statistics of birth, the number of new cases of AIDS and the length of waiting lists for hip operations, for example. In addition many articles will assume they are familiar with **confidence intervals** and related **significance tests**. Clearly lack of some basic statistical training will severely curtail a clinician's ability to evaluate critically much of the medical literature.

However, a knowledge of statistics is not only relevant in enabling the clinician to appraise the medical literature sensibly. Statistical issues are at least implicit in virtually all clinical practice, from the taking of routine observations to the evaluation of competing treatments. To see why, it will be helpful to direct our interest to a number of key clinical problems.

1.4 KEY PROBLEMS

Display 1.1 lists a series of five key questions which arise in both routine clinical practice and in clinical research. These questions will be used to motivate the rest of the book.

1	What is it?	The problem of diagnosis
2	How bad is it?	The problem of measurement
3	How common is it?	The estimation of prevalence
4	What caused it?	The search for associations
5	Can we treat it?	The evaluation of therapies

DISPLAY 1.1 The five key problems

What is it and how bad is it?

Clinicians are routinely involved in taking measurements and making observations on patients, and using the results to try to decide both what illness a patient is suffering from and how badly. The normal temperature for adults is, for example, 98.4°F and the normal blood pressure is 120/80 mm Hg. A family doctor finding a patient's temperature is 100°F or a blood pressure of 160/100 mm Hg, uses his/her experience to judge whether the values are far enough away from the normal values to suggest that the patient may have a problem. Underpinning this procedure is the realization that some departure from the normal values is to be expected even amongst patients who are well. Not all temperatures different from 98.4°F indicate that the patient may be ill, only those outside (either higher or lower) some limiting values. The family doctor will have in mind limits based on her previous experience, but it is very likely that this is combined with an appreciation of statistical principles, which suggest that measurements lying more than two standard deviations from the normal value are those that may give most cause for concern (see Chapter 4).

If the family doctor considers that the measurements made on her patient are abnormal, she may decide that some action is necessary. For the raised temperature this may be nothing more than prescribing two aspirins and a day in bed, based on a diagnosis that the patient simply has a cold. For the high blood pressure, she may consider that further and more detailed investigations are necessary before making her diagnosis. Here these might involve objective laboratory tests for the level of metabolites and other compounds in the patient's blood or urine. In other cases a patient's condition may call for more subjective measurements, such as an assessment of their pain, anxiety or depression.

There are several questions one can ask about the measurement process and the various measuring instruments. Is the device actually measuring what is intended, and how well is it doing it? Do competing instruments measure the desired characteristic equally well? Could one method (a cheaper one, perhaps) be used instead of another without significant loss of information? What is the ***precision (reliability)*** of a particular method of measurement? And so on. These questions of precision and reliability will be discussed in Chapter 3.

After having made a number of routine measurements, and if necessary a number that are less routine, the clinician will finally make a diagnosis of the patient's condition. You do not have to be a clinician to appreciate the problems of medical diagnosis, in particular to realize that the diagnostic process is not infallible. A patient exhibiting symptoms of severe chest pain and/or back pain and breathlessness might, for example, be diagnosed as suffering from a pulmonary embolism, since from past experience these symptoms have been associated with patients having this condition. But the correct diagnosis may be different; perhaps the patient had lifted a heavy load before running to the doctor's surgery. . .

The problem of diagnosis is to select the diagnostic category that is most likely given the characteristics of the patient's illness. Essentially this involves the statistical concept of probability, particularly conditional probability and the combination of such quantities using Bayes' theorem. These are all the subjects of Chapter 2.

How common is it?

One of the most important questions about disease and illness in a public health context is 'How widespread is it in the community?'. Clearly the answer to this question is vital in considering the rational allocation of health service resources. Readers are likely to be familiar with attempts to predict the future number of people with AIDS, or perhaps the number of elderly patients who will suffer from dementia. Such predictions are needed, for example, in order to assess the likely service needs in the twenty-first century.

Knowing how common a particular complaint is also has implications for diagnosis. Suppose, for example, a physician in the United Kingdom is faced with a shivering patient with a high temperature. In the absence of further information, the most likely diagnoses are flu or the common cold, since they are very common in Britain and are known to lead to the observed symptoms. A doctor in Ghana, however, confronted with a patient with the same symptoms, is perhaps more likely to diagnose malaria. In Africa in general, and Ghana in particular, malaria is still a common disease. In Britain, however, the disease is fortunately very rare, and without other evidence a diagnosis of malaria is very likely to be wrong.

Answering the question 'How common is it?' is not always as straightforward as it might first appear. There are two ways of measuring disease frequency, namely the **incidence** of the disease and its **prevalence**. The first of these says something about the number of new cases of a disease appearing during some fixed period of time. The prevalence of a disease is the number of individuals with the disease either at some fixed time (point prevalence) or during a given time interval (period prevalence). Incidence measures the rate of appearance of an illness and is therefore a measure of *risk* of the illness (see Chapter 5). Both incidence and prevalence are indicators of *morbidity*. If the illness is life-threatening, we may wish to look at the proportion of people who die through contracting the illness. These provide estimates of rates of *mortality*. The role of prevalence (or incidence) in the diagnostic process will be discussed in Chapter 2, its estimation will be discussed in Chapter 4.

What caused it?

The most important aim of many medical investigations is to seek the answer to this question, or perhaps, more realistically, to the question: 'What may have caused it?'. As in diagnosis, there will always be some level of doubt and uncertainty—we can never be sure that we have ruled out all possible competing causes. In some cases the search for a cause may involve little more than some intelligent detective work. In March 1991, for example, Somerset Health Authority's department of public health was informed of a mysterious 'slapped face' rash at one of the holiday sites in the area. Gunnell (1992) describes how the cause of the outbreak—irritation from washing powder in inadequately-rinsed bed linen—was tracked down with the help of an experiment that compared the outcome for people sleeping with new sheets and pillows with those using linen which had been laundered on the site.

Usually the search for possible causes is much more difficult than in the above illustration. This is the province of *epidemiology*. Many epidemiological studies receive wide publicity since they involve issues of major concern to the general public. Well-known examples include the search for the link between cigarette smoking and lung cancer, the possible influence of nuclear radiation on childhood leukaemia, and the effects of promiscuity on the incidence of sexually-transmitted diseases. Here we illustrate some of the problems by reference to work on the possible association between oral contraceptive use by women and subsequent development of breast cancer. The following is taken from a well-known Sunday newspaper.

A study showing an increase in breast cancer among women who use the pill is likely to spark a new scare when it is released this week.

The study from Sweden shows that women who use the pill long-term before the age of 25 are at greater risk of the disease later in life. . . .

Another study which contradicts the Swedish findings will be published this week. It will appear in the *British Medical Journal*. It comes from New Zealand and suggests that the use of the pill is not a risk factor in breast cancer.

Researchers in New Zealand can point for support to a vast American study in the *New England Journal of Medicine*. This compares 4711 women with breast cancer to 4670 without the disease and showed no increased risk. It was found that 1756 of those with the disease had used the contraceptive pill while 1699 of those without had also used it. The difference was found to be insignificant in statistical terms.

The Observer, September 1986

Note that the different studies reach different conclusions, a not infrequent finding in epidemiological research where the effects under investigation can be relatively subtle. Epidemiological problems are the subject of Chapter 5.

Can we treat it?

Of great concern to all clinicians faced with a suffering patient is 'Can we help?', or more specifically, 'Can we cure the illness?' Indeed the same question must have been critical to all those practising medicine through the ages, from the African witch-doctor faced with the ailing son of the chief, to Henry VIII's physician confronting the king after he had suffered a riding accident.

In the past, evidence for the efficacy of various remedies would have come from the clinician's personal experience and from anecdotal evidence provided by others. Often the methods were backed by little more than faith. We may smugly look back at the days of blood-letting and think that similarly unsubstantiated procedures would not be used now. But is this really true? Many so-called therapies are never properly evaluated and many patients of the present authors' age have had so-called vestigial organs (such as tonsils and the appendix) surgically removed during their childhood for apparently no valid reason.

The preferred way of evaluating competing therapies is through the use of a carefully designed experiment—known as the **controlled clinical trial**. The controlled trial has a surprisingly recent history, the first, which took place just after the Second World War, involving an evaluation of streptomycin in the treatment of pulmonary tuberculosis. Since then they have become commonplace and the rationale for their use is discussed in detail in Chapter 6. Well-known examples are trials of the Salk polio vaccine in the 1950s and recent trials of AZT (azidothymidine) for the treatment and prevention of AIDS in HIV-infected patients. The design and analysis of clinical trials are discussed in the final chapter.

1.5 SUMMARY

You may still not be entirely sympathetic with Florence Nightingale's enthusiasm concerning the use of statistics, but we hope that we might have alerted you at least to its vital importance in both clinical practice and medical research. As a clinician you will certainly become a consumer of statistical information, and it is important that you understand the language and can make critical attempts at its evaluation. If you go into medical research you are likely to also become a producer of statistical information as well as a consumer. Here, for both scientific and ethical reasons, there will be an obligation placed on you to use statistical methods in an appropriate way. Ignorance is not a valid excuse for the abuse of statistical information—particularly when it can lead to patients being exposed to useless and potentially harmful 'therapies'—or to a truly beneficial treatment being abandoned because of defective trials of its efficacy.

Having, we hope, convinced you of the need to learn about medical statistics, we now need to develop your interest and not frighten you off with perhaps boring and unnecessarily technical detail. The aim of this book is to demonstrate that the statistical expertise most needed by the majority of medical students and practising clinicians *can* be learnt relatively painlessly. The philosophy behind the present authors' approach is that the learner will be more highly motivated if the statistical methods are presented as ways of solving clinically important problems. Hence the five key questions in Display 1.1. The following five chapters are each based on the provision of the answers to these problems.

By the end of the book we hope that you will have moved well way from the attitude summarized both by Disraeli's well known 'lies, damned lies and statistics' and by the following quotation from Chamberlain (1991):

> Doctors are mostly literate, but are commonly innumerate. We are largely ignorant and frightened of the safe and helpful use of figures because we have never been taught to understand them properly. In consequence we often try to dismiss them, believing that they are used during medical debate in a biased fashion to support the arguments of the proponents but are put to one side as non-relevant or non-significant by the opponents. This is a head-in-the-sand attitude as statistics are extremely helpful in providing evidence of changes.

FURTHER READING

At the end of each chapter in the book will be a selection of references for further reading. It goes without saying that we are expecting you to continue reading the remaining chapters of the present book! Many readers, however, will wish to go further. Here we give two papers which have a similar philosophy to the present text:

Evidence-Based Medicine Working Group (1992). Evidence-based medicine. A new approach to teaching the practice of medicine. *Journal of the American Medical Association* **268**, 2420–5.

Oxman, A.D., Sackett, D.L. and Guyatt, G.H. (1993). Users' guides to the medical literature. 1. How to get started. *Journal of the American Medical Association* **270**, 2093–5.

Diagnosis, Probability and Sampling

2

2.1 INTRODUCTION

Suppose that an overweight middle-aged man consults you concerning chest pains. During your interview with him you discover that he is suffering from stress at work and has a history of hypertension (high blood pressure). The temptation may be to diagnose heart disease but there may be other possibilities. After examining the results of laboratory and other tests you requested to assist you in your decision, how would you use the resulting information to come to a diagnosis? You might, of course, rely heavily on your previous experience and clinical knowledge but formally this problem involves the manipulation (combination) and interpretation of *probabilities*. The question is:

'Given the patient's symptoms and diagnostic test results, what is the probability of heart disease?'

To illustrate what might be involved in this process let us consider a rather simpler example. Suppose that you work in a coronary care unit. All patients under the age of 70 who are suspected of having a myocardial infarction (heart attack) within the previous 48 hours are admitted to this unit. Some of these patients actually have had a heart attack and it is therefore appropriate that they should be treated within the unit. Others, however, will not have had a heart attack (but may be suffering from another illness—severe indigestion, for example) and could be transferred to another part of your hospital or simply discharged. It is vital that you distinguish between the two types of patient as soon as possible and as accurately as possible: discharging a heart attack patient with the advice to take some antacid tablets may have very serious consequences (both for the patient and yourself as the responsible clinician!).

Suppose that the results of a laboratory test are available to help with your diagnostic decision (measurement of a serum enzyme such as creatine kinase, for example, where raised levels are associated with heart attacks). The test results can be said to be 'positive' or 'negative' depending on whether the measured quantity is greater or less than some previously specified threshold and the patient's true status is either 'infarct' or 'no infarct'. In this simple but clinically unrealistic example (in practice the results from many tests would be available), the problem becomes one of calculating the probability of the patient having had a heart attack given the nature of the test result. Using data from Smith (1967), it is discussed in considerable detail by Sackett *et al.* (1991).

Both examples above indicate that the main statistical concept underlying the diagnostic process is that of probability. It is this and the related concept of odds that are the subjects of the next section.

2.2 PROBABILITIES AND ODDS

There is no completely satisfactory explanation of probability. Probability is one of those elusive concepts that virtually everyone talks about, but which is almost impossible to define adequately. Most aspects of life, however, involve some probabilistic statements, and medicine is no exception. What is the probability that a patient with AIDS will live for a further year? What is the probability that an individual taking daily vitamin C will have fewer colds than individuals not taking the compound? What is the probability, given the outcome of a set of diagnostic tests, that the patient in front of you is suffering from tuberculosis of the lung?

Probability statements are quantified on a scale ranging from 0 to 1. An event with probability of zero cannot happen; an event with a probability of one is certain to happen. When someone assigns a probability to an event it is a statement of their degree of belief that it will happen—the higher the probability the more likely the event is thought to be. A probability is somewhat similar to a fraction, proportion or percentage. An event with a probability of one fifth (1/5 or 0.2) means that there is a 1 in 5 or 20% chance of it happening. Equivalently, we can express this chance in the form of **odds**: the odds against the event are 4 to 1 (or 4:1), or, alternatively, the odds in favour are 1 to 4. It is customary (particularly in arithmetical calculations) to drop the 'to 1' from statements about odds of the form '*a* to 1' and just write the odds as '*a*'. (Note that this *only* applies when the odds are expressed as '*a* to 1' and not '*a* to *b*', for example.) So, if we say that the odds in favour of a given disease are 3.5 or 0.75, we are using the numbers as an abbreviation of 3.5 to 1 (or 3.5:1) and 0.75 to 1 (or 0.75:1), respectively. The gamblers amongst you should already be familiar with the manipulation of odds. Others will easily gain the required familiarity with practice.

It is not necessary to have a detailed knowledge of the mathematics of probabilities or odds to understand the methods of statistical inference to be discussed in the following chapters. It is useful, however, to be familiar with some of the simple rules for combining probabilities and, in particular, the use of *conditional probabilities* and a technique called *Bayes' theorem*.

Assigning and combining probabilities

As mentioned above, there is no single completely satisfactory definition of probability, but one that is often used is that the probability of some specific event is the proportion of times that the event occurs in a large series of observations. So, for example, if amongst 100 000 births, 51 000 were boys, then the probability of a boy, usually written P(boy), would be represented by the fraction 51 000/100 000 = 0.51. Similarly, the probability of being a girl is 0.49. This *long-term relative frequency* method of assigning probabilities is sufficient for most of our needs. In this example, the events of interest are 'being a boy' or 'being a girl'. The word 'event' seems a bit abstract, but can mean 'suffers from illness X', 'dies', 'recovers', 'has positive blood test', 'has high blood pressure', 'is anxious', and so on. It is any feature or characteristic that can vary from one observation to another, or from one patient to another. (A more technical term that we shall use occasionally is *random variable*.) If something is fixed or immutable (the truth or otherwise of a scientific theory or hypothesis, or the existence of God)—that is, *not* a random variable—then it makes no sense to assign probability statements to it. Some people (confusingly called *Bayesians* from the way in which they interpret the use of Bayes' theorem) do assign probabilities to the truth of theories, however, but this use of the concept would not be consistent with our use of the long-term relative frequency definition of probability. We will not use probability in this way.

When probabilities have been assigned to events it is often required to find the probability associated with some combination of these events. If we know, for example, that P(boy) = 0.51 and P(girl) = 0.49, what is the probability that in a family of two children, the older is a girl and the younger a boy? There are basically two relatively simple rules for combining probabilities.

(a) The probabilities of either of two events   If A and B are two events with probabilities P(A) and P(B), what is the probability of either A or B occurring? The required probability is simply the **sum** of the separate probabilities, provided the events are **mutually exclusive** (i.e. they cannot both happen together). So if, for example, the probability of an individual being blood group O is 0.46, and that for blood group B is 0.08, then the probability of being either group O or group B is 0.54 (0.46 + 0.08).

From above, we have P(boy) = 0.51 and P(girl) = 0.49, so using the addition rule the probability of a boy or a girl is 0.51 + 0.49 = 1.00. It must *always* be the case that the probabilities of all possible outcomes must add up to one, since one of the possibilities must occur. Suppose, for example, that a particular symptom can only be caused by one of three mutually exclusive illnesses (that is the illnesses cannot occur together). Then the probability of illness A plus the probability of illness B plus the probability of illness C must sum to one, otherwise another possible cause of the symptom exists.

(b) Probability of both of two events   If A and B are two events with probabilities P(A) and P(B), what is the probability that both occur? Here the answer is that, provided the two events are **independent**, P(A and B) is simply the **product** of the separate probabilities. Statistical independence means that the outcome of one event tells us nothing about the other event. So, for example, for two unrelated individuals the probability that they are both blood group B is 0.08 × 0.08 = 0.0064. If two events are *not* independent then this simple form of the multiplication rule does not apply and we have to consider conditional probabilities.

Conditional probability

The concept of statistical independence is linked to that of **conditional probability**, the probability of an event occurring *given* that another event has already occurred (or conditional on the occurrence of another event). We write the conditional probability of B occurring given that A has occurred as $P(B|A)$. Note that the vertical line '|' does not indicate division (this is indicated by the oblique stroke '/'). As an example consider colour blindness in humans. Here the probability of a person being colour blind, given that the person is male, is about 0.05; the corresponding probability, given that the person is female, is only 0.0025.

The probability that two non-independent events occur together can be written in terms of conditional probabilities as shown in Display 2.1. In words, the probability of both events A and B occurring is the product of $P(A)$ and $P(B|A)$. It is also the product of $P(B)$ and $P(A|B)$.

Conditional probabilities are particularly important in describing the performance of those diagnostic tests which can yield either a positive or negative result, the former suggesting that the patient has the condition under investigation. One such test was introduced earlier, the use of serum creatine kinase (CK) as an indicator of probable heart failure. Another example considered in the exercises at the end of this chapter involves the use of mammography in the diagnosis of breast cancer. In each case the test will suggest whether the patient is ill or well, and in each case the patient will actually have the condition or not.

The first conditional probability to consider is the probability of the test being positive given that the disease is present, for example, $P(CK+|infarct)$. This is known as the **sensitivity** of a test. The **specificity** of a test, on the other hand, is the probability of the test being negative given that the disease is absent, $P(CK-|no\ infarct)$, for example. So, sensitivity measures the ability of a test to correctly

Probability of A given B = $P(A|B)$
Probability of B given A = $P(B|A)$
Probability of A and B   = $P(A\ and\ B)$

$P(A\ and\ B) = P(A) \times P(B|A)$
$P(A\ and\ B) = P(B) \times P(A|B)$

DISPLAY 2.1 Conditional probability

identify a person with the condition (often called a *case*); and specificity measures the ability of the test to correctly identify a non-case. The calculation of sensitivity and specificity in general is illustrated in Display 2.2 and specifically for some data on the creatine test in Display 2.3.

An alternative way of looking at the performance of a test is in terms of the types of errors made. A *false positive*, for example, occurs when a positive test result appears in a non-case (CK+ when the patient has not had a heart attack). A *false negative* is a negative test result for a subject who, in fact, is a case (CK− when the patient has had a heart attack). The corresponding probabilities are referred to as the *false positive rate* and the *false negative rate*, respectively. Two other conditional probabilities of great importance are the test's *positive predictive value* (PPV) and its *negative predictive value* (NPV). The former is the conditional probability that the subject has the disease given a positive test result (the

---

(a) Counts:

True diagnosis

Test result		Positive	Negative	Total
	Positive	a	b	$a+b$
	Negative	c	d	$c+d$
	Total	$a+c$	$b+d$	$N=a+b+c+d$

(b) Definitions:

In terms of the counts a (true positives), b (false positives), c (false negatives) and d (true negatives):

Sensitivity	$= a/(a+c)$
Specificity	$= d/(b+d)$
False positive rate	$= b/(b+d)$
False negative rate	$= c/(a+c)$
Positive predictive value	$= a/(a+b)$
Negative predictive value	$= d/(c+d)$

DISPLAY 2.2 Characteristics of diagnostic tests

		True diagnosis (heart attack)		
		Positive	Negative	Total
Test result	Positive	215	16	231
	Negative	15	114	129
	Total	230	130	360

Sensitivity   = 215/230 = 0.93 (93%)
Specificity   = 114/130 = 0.88 (88%)
False positive rate   = 16/130 = 0.12 (12%)
False negative rate   = 15/230 = 0.07 (7%)
Positive predictive value   = 215/231 = 0.93 (93%)
Negative predictive value   = 114/129 = 0.88 (88%)

DISPLAY 2.3 Characteristics of the creatine kinase test (Smith, 1967)

proportion of people with positive test results who are, in fact, cases: P(infarct|CK+), for example), and the latter is the conditional probability that the subject is disease-free given a negative test result (the proportion of people with negative test results who are, in fact, not cases: P(no infarct|CK−), for example). In terms of making decisions, these are the two key probabilities used in making diagnoses. Again, the terms are illustrated in Displays 2.2 and 2.3.

Bayes' theorem

In the 18th century an Englishman, Thomas Bayes, wrote an essay on probability, part of which gave rise to an extremely important method of calculating probabilities taking account of new information. Bayes' theorem, as the method is now known, plays a key role in recent developments in automated and computer-assisted diagnosis and pertains directly to the logic underlying a medical diagnosis. The formulae for Bayes' theorem are given in Display 2.4, but perhaps greater insight into its utility can be achieved by means of a number of examples.

Returning to Display 2.3, this presents data on the relationship between heart attacks and the creatine kinase (CK) test. The sensitivity of the test is 93%; its specificity is 88%. Its PPV can be

Consider a disease (D) which can either be present (D+) or absent (D−). Similarly a diagnostic test (T) can be either positive (T+) or negative (T−).

$$P(T+ \text{ and } D+) \quad = P(T+) \times P(D+|T+)$$
$$= P(D+) \times P(T+|D+)$$

Equating these two expressions:

$$P(T+) \times P(D+|T+) \quad = P(D+) \times P(T+|D+)$$

Therefore, dividing both sides by $P(T+)$:

$$P(D+|T+) \quad = P(D+) \times P(T+|D+)/P(T+)$$

Posterior probability = Prior probability × Likelihood

DISPLAY 2.4 Bayes' theorem

ascertained directly from the table, and is found to be 93%. Similarly the NPV is 88%. Alternatively, the PPV can be calculated indirectly through the use of Bayes' theorem as:

PPV = Sensitivity × Prevalence/P(Test+)

$$= (215/230) \times (230/260)/(231/360)$$

$$= 215/231, \text{ or } 93\%, \text{ as before.}$$

The ratio, Sensitivity/P(Test+) is known as the *likelihood* of disease given a positive test result, and another way of expressing Bayes' theorem using this term is:

$$P(D+|T+) = P(D+) \times \text{Likelihood}$$

The conditional probability on the left-hand side of this equation is usually known as the *posterior probability* and the probability term on the right-hand side of the equation as the *prior probability* so that Bayes' theorem can also be put in the form:

Posterior probability = Prior probability × Likelihood

The ratio P(Test+|Disease−)/P(Test+), equivalent to (1 − Specificity)/P(Test+), is the likelihood of no disease given a positive test result. The *likelihood ratio* (LR) is the ratio of the likelihood of disease given a positive test result to the likelihood of no disease given a positive test result. That is:

Likelihood ratio (LR) = Sensitivity/(1 − Specificity)

Notice that the term P(Test+) was common to both likelihoods and therefore disappears when the ratio is calculated. The use of the likelihood ratio enables us to use a version of Bayes' theorem involving odds rather than probabilities. That is:

Posterior odds = Prior odds × Likelihood ratio

The likelihood ratio is a single number that can be used to characterize a diagnostic or screening test (although it is often useful to know both the test's sensitivity and its specificity). It is particularly useful because it is not dependent on the proportion of cases or positive test results in the population (unlike the likelihood, itself, which is dependent on P(Test+)). Note that the above odds are those in favour of disease (unlike gambling on horses where the odds against winning are those usually quoted). In the above creatine kinase-heart attack example the likelihood ratio is given by ((215/230)/(16/130)) and the posterior odds are therefore:

$$\text{Posterior odds} = (230/130) \times [(215/230)/(16/130)]$$

$$= 215/16$$

$$= 13.4375$$

As odds = probability/(1 − probability) it follows from simple algebra that probability = odds/(1 + odds), and

$$\text{Posterior probability} = 13.4375/(1 + 13.4375)$$

$$= 0.93, \text{ or } 93\% \text{ (as before)}$$

Now, to summarize the procedure, we can consider a final example based on the work of Sivak and Wormser (1986) and also discussed by Strike (1991). This example involves the screening of blood donors for evidence of HIV infection using a simple, but fallible, antibody test. Let us assume that the true prevalence of HIV infection in blood donors is 1 per 1000 (0.1%), corresponding to a prior odds of 1 to 999 (almost exactly the same as odds of 1 to 1000 or 0.001, so we will use 0.001). Let the sensitivity of the antibody test be 85% and its specificity be 99%. That is,

$$P(Ab+/HIV+) = 0.85$$

and $\qquad P(Ab+/HIV-) = 0.01 \text{ (i.e. } 1 - 0.99)$

Hence

$$\text{Likelihood ratio} = \text{Sensitivity}/(1 - \text{Specificity})$$

$$= 0.85/0.01$$

$$= 85$$

What are the posterior odds of HIV infection given a positive antibody test result? These are given by the product of the prior odds and the likelihood ratio:

$$\text{Posterior odds} = 0.001 \times 85$$

$$= 0.085$$

The posterior probability is $0.085/(1 + 0.085) = 0.078$. So, even if a blood donor is apparently antibody positive, the probability of being HIV+ is still less than 1 in 10. You may find this low value quite surprising. It is this low, of course, because of the very small number of blood donors with HIV infection. If, however, the population being screened were composed of heroine addicts, then the prior odds would be much greater. For the sake of argument, let the prior odds be 1 to 10. Now the posterior odds are 8.5 to 1, corresponding to a posterior probability of about 89%. So, your diagnostic decision is not only determined by the efficiency of the test (its sensitivity and specificity) but is vitally dependent on a sensible estimate of the prevalence of the disease or illness in the population of interest (your *target population*—see next section). Prevalence estimation will be considered in detail in Chapter 4. Here we will consider how you might estimate the sensitivity and specificity of a test or, alternatively, evaluate the quality of published estimates of these characteristics.

2.3 POPULATIONS, TARGET POPULATIONS AND SAMPLES

As in other areas that we shall consider in later chapters, the primary aim in the investigation of the properties of a diagnostic test is to generalize the results from a sample of individuals, typically patients, to the population in which we are interested. This population might be a particular community, general practice or health clinic attenders, drug addicts, people with suspected heart failure, pregnant women, and so on. The method of selection of the individuals to be used in the investigation is of considerable importance for the production of valid test results and conclusions. In general, the most important requirement is to obtain a sample which is truly representative of the population of interest (that is the *target population*). We need to ensure that the *sampled population* is the same as, or at least very close to, the target population. Unless this can be achieved, any inferences that we draw about the population are likely to be suspect.

Consider, for example, a study involving the evaluation of the creatine kinase test for heart failure as mentioned in the previous section. Suppose the investigator responsible for recruiting patients works in a large university hospital, and chooses 50 patients admitted to the hospital's coronary care unit. At the end of the investigation, the research team's aim is to draw some conclusion about both the likely efficacy of the diagnostic test for the 50 particular patients in the sample, and when used on suspected coronary patients in general. Any such conclusion, however, would need to be tempered by the considerations of what possible *selective factors* and *biases* distinguish the population actually sampled, namely all admissions to the coronary care unit at this particular university hospital, from the target population of all patients with suspected heart failure. Two such selective factors come immediately to mind. First, not all patients with a suspected myocardial infarction will be referred to the unit. There might be a considerable proportion of patients who are not recognized by the family doctor, for example, as probably having had a heart attack. Such patients could not have been chosen to take part in the study because of the manner in which the sample was selected. Second, even amongst those patients whose suspected heart condition is severe enough to require hospital treatment, those admitted to a specialist coronary care unit in a university hospital are likely to be the more serious or complicated cases. For these reasons, it may be completely misleading to draw conclusions about the efficacy of the test for all patients with a suspected myocardial infarction from the information gathered from this particular sample.

Even having ensured that the appropriate population is being sampled, however, it is equally important that the actual sample is drawn in an objective and unbiased way. Haphazard samples, or samples selected on the basis of being easy to collect, are rarely representative of the population. It is important that the investigator does not select patients for laboratory tests on the basis of the symptoms or other characteristics of the patient (this situation is clearly different to routine clinical practice in which the doctor will obviously use subjective clinical judgements all the time). It would be invalid, for example, to select two sub-samples of patients—one sample of those who have almost certainly had a heart attack as seen by the severity of their symptoms and another who almost certainly have not (i.e. excluding the confusing patients in the middle). There are now several well-established methods for selecting a sample to avoid subjective biases. Most have as their basis the concept of a *random* or *probability sample*, in which every individual or patient in the population of interest is selected (or not) through the use of a clearly described random mechanism (as in tossing coins or throwing dice, for example). In the simplest example, a *simple random sampling scheme*, each possible *sample* is equally likely. The corollary of this is that each patient has an equal probability of being included in the sample. This sampling method, and others, will be discussed further in Chapter 4.

2.4 SAMPLING VARIATION

Let us assume that we wish to estimate the sensitivity of the creatine kinase test. We obtain a sample of 10 patients who are known to have suffered from a heart attack within, say, 48 hours of testing. We find that eight of the 10 patients are CK+. So our estimate of sensitivity is 80% (note that what is being estimated here is a proportion). It does not need any great knowledge of statistics to realize that we cannot be very confident in this estimate. If we were to test another sample of 10 similar patients we might find that only half of them provide positive test results, or even that all of them do. This is an example of *sampling variation*. It should also be fairly obvious to you that if we were to estimate the sensitivity of the diagnostic test using a larger sample of patients then we should get a more dependable value, one that on repeated sampling would be less variable. How do we measure the dependability of our estimates, and how large a sample is needed in order to get an estimate that is dependable enough? Before providing an answer to these questions it is of interest to examine an example of sampling variation in a little more detail. This can be done very simply using computer-simulated samples and Display 2.5 provides a table of

68	64	.76	74	76	82	66	80	72
72	72	74	60	74	76	78	74	72
74	74	72	70	54	74	72	62	76
76	84	82	82	70	80	82	72	68
72	66	72	60	72	72	74	76	66
70	70	72	66	76	72	78	70	74
70	76	74	66	60	68	62	66	76
80	72	68	66	76	70	60	82	76
64	76	68	58	72	70	82	70	76
74	78	72	78	70	82	70	76	68
70	84	70	84	78	62	74	66	64
78	74	72	68	66	68	56	56	74
70	68	68	66	76	68	78	68	72
66	60	68	76	62	62	68	74	58
76	76	76	76	74	64	76	76	78
80	72	68	68	66	66	76	56	66
72	76	66	70	74	70			

DISPLAY 2.5 Computer simulated test data (sensitivity as percentages)

sensitivity estimates obtained from 150 simulated samples each with 50 'patients', where the true value of the sensitivity is 70% (this is built into the simulations).

As it stands, Display 2.5 is a bit difficult to take in. We can search for particularly low, or particularly high, values and perhaps get some idea of a typical value; but the values really need to be rearranged in some way in order to make them more easily digested. One way of doing this is to sort the data so that the lowest value is the first entry, the next from the bottom the second entry, and so on all the way up to the highest value (alternatively, they could be ordered starting with the highest and proceeding to the lowest). The rearranged table is shown in Display 2.6. Counts of identical values can then be made and the data further summarized by a table of relative frequencies (Display 2.7). This table is an example of what is generally known as a *sampling distribution*—it shows, in this case, how the sensitivity estimates are distributed in repeated samples. A graphical representation of the data, known as a *histogram*, is shown in Display 2.8. Here the number of sensitivity estimates with a particular value is represented by a rectangle of appropriate length. (Both sampling distributions and histograms are discussed in more detail in Chapter 4.) You can see from the histogram that the values

54	56	56	56	58	58	60	60	60
60	60	62	62	62	62	62	64	64
64	64	66	66	66	66	66	66	66
66	66	66	66	66	66	66	66	68
68	68	68	68	68	68	68	68	68
68	68	68	68	68	68	70	70	70
70	70	70	70	70	70	70	70	70
70	70	70	70	72	72	72	72	72
72	72	72	72	72	72	72	72	72
72	72	72	72	72	72	74	74	74
74	74	74	74	74	74	74	74	74
74	74	74	74	74	76	76	76	76
76	76	76	76	76	76	76	76	76
76	76	76	76	76	76	76	76	76
76	76	78	78	78	78	78	78	78
78	80	80	80	80	82	82	82	82
82	82	82	84	84	84			

DISPLAY 2.6 Sorted sensitivity estimates (from Display 2.5)

Value	Frequency	Relative frequency (%)	Cumulative frequency (%)
54	1	0.7	0.7
56	3	2.0	2.7
58	2	1.3	4.0
60	5	3.3	7.3
62	5	3.3	10.7
64	4	2.7	13.3
66	15	10.0	23.3
68	16	10.7	34.0
70	16	10.7	44.7
72	20	13.3	58.0
74	17	11.3	69.3
76	24	16.0	85.3
78	8	5.3	90.7
80	4	2.7	93.3
82	7	4.7	98.0
84	3	2.0	100.0
TOTAL	150	100.0	

DISPLAY 2.7 Frequency distributions for data in Display 2.5

Count Value

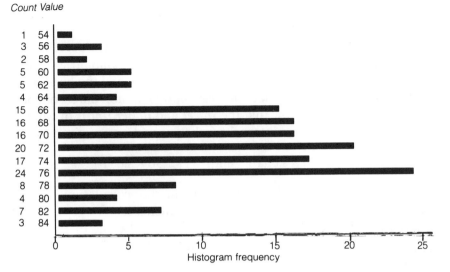

DISPLAY 2.8 Histogram of sensitivity estimates

are more or less symmetrically distributed about the true sensitivity value of 70%. The average value (the *arithmetic mean* obtained by adding together all 150 entries in the table and dividing by 150) is, in fact, 71.3%. The middle value (the *median*) is 72%. The smallest value is 54% and the largest is 84% giving a total *range* (the arithmetic difference between maximum and minimum values) of 30%. So, even with a sample size as large as 50 patients the variation between repeated samples is quite considerable.

In practice, of course, we do not have the luxury of looking at sampling variability directly by repeated sampling as in Display 2.5. We just have a single estimate of a test's sensitivity (74%, for example) and a knowledge of the size of the tested sample (50, say). How can we assess the dependability of our estimate? This is done by calculating what is known as the *standard error* of the estimate and using this standard error to determine a *confidence interval*. The arithmetic is very simple. For any proportion, P, estimated using a sample of size N, the standard error (s.e.) is given by:

$$\text{s.e.}(P) = \text{sqrt}[P(1 - P)/N]$$

Where 'sqrt' means 'the square root of'. If we work with percentages rather than proportions, then the standard error is:

$$\text{s.e.}(P) = \text{sqrt}[P(100 - P)/N]$$

So, for example, an estimate of 74%, based on a sample of 50 patients, has a standard error of 6.2%.

Now, if the sampling distribution of a proportion (or percentage) follows a **Normal distribution** (a completely symmetrical bell-shaped curve—see Chapter 4 for further details), and the histogram in Display 2.8 suggests that this assumption is not unreasonable, then it is possible to show that the **lower** and **upper limits** of what is called a 95% confidence interval for the proportion are given by:

$$P - 1.96 \times s.e.(P) \quad \text{and} \quad P + 1.96 \times s.e.(P)$$

respectively. (In most cases the '1.96' in this calculation can be replaced by '2' without any serious consequences!)

When, as in the above example, the observed value of P is 74% the corresponding lower and upper limits of the 95% confidence interval are:

$$74 - 1.96 \times 6.2 = 61.8 \quad \text{and} \quad 74 + 1.96 \times 6.2 = 86.15$$

The 95% confidence interval is usually represented in the form (61.8, 86.15)—the lower and upper limits are separated by a comma, and both together are then surrounded by a pair of parentheses. Display 2.9 provides 95% confidence interval estimates for each of the 150 computer-simulated examples in Display 2.5. Note that this interval varies randomly from one sample to another. It is another example of a random variable.

The calculations in this case are easy, but we now have to consider a little more carefully what the term 'confidence interval' really means. How does percentage confidence relate to probability, itself expressed as a percentage? We start by emphasizing that under constant laboratory conditions the true, but unknown, sensitivity is a fixed value. It is *not* a random variable. If we regard a probability as a long-term relative frequency on repeated sampling we cannot then make a probability statement about the sensitivity of the test (or any other population quantity or **parameter** that is being estimated). It is our sample **statistic** (the observed value of the sensitivity in a given sample, or the confidence interval determined from that sample) which is the random variable. It does, therefore, make sense to ask 'What is the probability that the calculated confidence interval includes the true, but unknown, value?'. This is equivalent to asking about the proportion of times confidence intervals from repeated samples actually contain the unknown value being estimated. For a

(55.07, 80.93)	(71.35, 92.65)	(48.55, 75.45)
(59.55, 84.45)	(46.42, 73.58)	(46.42, 73.58)
(61.84, 86.16)	(52.87, 79.13)	(71.35, 92.65)
(64.16, 87.84)	(52.87, 79.13)	(57.30, 82.70)
(59.55, 84.45)	(52.87, 79.13)	(61.84, 86.16)
(57.30, 82.70)	(44.32, 71.68)	(42.24, 69.76)
(57.30, 82.70)	(66.52, 89.48)	(66.52, 89.48)
(68.91, 91.09)	(73.84, 94.16)	(55.07, 80.93)
(50.70, 77.30)	(55.07, 80.93)	(64.16, 87.84)
(61.84, 86.16)	(52.87, 79.13)	(64.16, 87.84)
(57.30, 82.70)	(64.16, 87.84)	(68.91, 91.09)
(66.52, 89.48)	(64.16, 87.84)	(61.84, 86.16)
(57.30, 82.70)	(55.07, 80.93)	(48.55, 75.45)
(52.87, 79.13)	(57.30, 82.70)	(59.55, 84.45)
(64.16, 87.84)	(64.16, 87.84)	(64.16, 87.84)
(68.91, 91.09)	(61.84, 86.16)	(57.30, 82.70)
(59.55, 84.45)	(40.19, 67.81)	(52.87, 79.13)
(50.70, 77.30)	(57.30, 82.70)	(71.35, 92.65)
(59.55, 84.45)	(59.55, 84.45)	(57.30, 82.70)
(61.84, 86.16)	(64.16, 87.84)	(64.16, 87.84)
(73.84, 94.16)	(46.42, 73.58)	(52.87, 79.13)
(52.87, 79.13)	(64.16, 87.84)	(42.24, 69.76)
(57.30, 82.70)	(59.55, 84.45)	(55.07, 80.93)
(64.16, 87.84)	(57.30, 82.70)	(61.84, 86.16)
(59.55, 84.45)	(66.52, 89.48)	(64.16, 87.84)
(64.16, 87.84)	(52.87, 79.13)	(42.24, 69.76)
(66.52, 89.48)	(64.16, 87.84)	(59.55, 84.45)
(73.84, 94.16)	(48.55, 75.45)	(59.55, 84.45)
(61.84, 86.16)	(61.84, 86.16)	(64.16, 87.84)
(55.07, 80.93)	(52.87, 79.13)	(55.07, 80.93)
(46.42, 73.58)	(61.84, 86.16)	(52.87, 79.13)
(64.16, 87.84)	(71.35, 92.65)	(61.84, 86.16)
(59.55, 84.45)	(64.16, 87.84)	(64.16, 87.84)
(64.16, 87.84)	(61.84, 86.16)	(64.16, 87.84)
(64.16, 87.84)	(68.91, 91.09)	(64.16, 87.84)
(61.84, 86.16)	(59.55, 84.45)	(55.07, 80.93)
(59.55, 84.45)	(59.55, 84.45)	(50.70, 77.30)
(71.35, 92.65)	(55.07, 80.93)	(61.84, 86.16)
(59.55, 84.45)	(57.30, 82.70)	(59.55, 84.45)
(59.55, 84.45)	(57.30, 82.70)	(44.32, 71.68)
(61.84, 86.16)	(71.35, 92.65)	(66.52, 89.48)
(55.07, 80.93)	(48.55, 75.45)	(52.87, 79.13)
(55.07, 80.93)	(55.07, 80.93)	
(59.55, 84.45)	(55.07, 80.93)	
(57.30, 82.70)	(48.55, 75.45)	
(59.55, 84.45)	(50.70, 77.30)	
(55.07, 80.93)	(52.87, 79.13)	
(55.07, 80.93)	(57.30, 82.70)	
(64.16, 87.84)	(52.87, 79.13)	
(55.07, 80.93)	(66.52, 89.48)	
(52.87, 79.13)	(59.55, 84.45)	
(61.84, 86.16)	(71.35, 92.65)	
(46.42, 73.58)	(61.84, 86.16)	
(57.30, 82.70)	(66.52, 89.48)	

DISPLAY 2.9 Approximate 95% confidence intervals from estimates in Display 2.5

95% confidence interval the answer is 19 times out of 20, or 95%. If we construct a 95% confidence interval each time we draw a sample and then claim that the true value of the unknown parameter is within this interval, then we will be wrong, on average, once in every 20 (or 5%) times. Display 2.9 illustrates this point. Each of the 150 samples has a corresponding confidence interval. We know in this case that the sensitivity of the diagnostic test is 70%. How often does this true value fall between the lower and upper limits of these confidence intervals? The answer is 136, or 90.7%. This is not quite the expected 95%. There are two possible reasons for this (and both are likely to hold). First, only 150 samples have been used—the proportion of our constructed confidence intervals that include the true sensitivity is itself only an estimate of the percentage confidence. Second, the assumption of Normality for the sampling distribution of the sensitivity estimates in Display 2.5 (see Display 2.8) is only an approximate one. The approximation, however, gets better with increasing sample size (see Section 4.5).

An estimate's standard error or, equivalently, the size of a confidence interval, is a measure of the *fallibility* of our estimate. The smaller the standard error (or the smaller the difference between lower and upper confidence limits) the better. A good estimate has a small standard error; a bad one a large standard error. A further property of a confidence interval is that if we want to be *more* confident then we have to accept a *larger* interval. A 99% confidence interval for a proportion, for example, is the observed value of the proportion plus or minus 2.58 standard errors. In the example considered above this leads to the interval (58.0, 90.0), which is seen to be somewhat wider than the 95% interval calculated earlier.

Finally, consider the situation where we are *planning* an evaluation of a laboratory test. In particular, we want to know how many patients to include in our sample. Suppose we have a rough idea of the test's sensitivity based on preliminary laboratory work and we think, for example, that it is about 75%. Suppose we want to estimate the test's sensitivity using a 95% confidence interval and want the size or width of this interval (that is, the difference between lower and upper confidence limits) to be no more than 10%. Again assuming that the sensitivity is normally distributed on repeated sampling, the width of a 95% confidence interval is plus or minus 1.96 standard errors. The standard error, in turn, is the square root of $P \times (100 - P)/N$, where P is the sensitivity of the test as a percentage and N is the sample size to be determined. This leads us to the following equality:

$$2 \times 1.96 \times \mathrm{sqrt}(P \times (100 - P)/N) = 10$$

where the initial '2' comes from 'plus or minus' 1.96 standard errors in the calculation of the 95% confidence interval. After substituting $P = 75\%$, this expression can then be re-arranged to give a solution for the unknown N. First we square both sides of the above expression:

$$4 \times 3.84 \times P \times (100 - P)/N = 100$$

Therefore

$$N = 4 \times 3.84 \times 75 \times 25/100$$
$$= 3.84 \times 75$$
$$= 288$$

2.5 CRITICAL APPRAISAL OF PUBLISHED TEST INFORMATION

The purpose of this section is to provide an overview of what has gone before, but to place the discussion in the context of you, as a potential user of test information, deciding on the utility (or otherwise) of a particular diagnostic test or screening instrument. It will take the form of a series of questions.

- Has there been an independent 'blind' comparison of the results of the test with a 'gold standard' of diagnosis? The gold standard might be the results of a detailed concurrent diagnostic examination; a follow-up examination when the picture will have been clarified from the natural history of the disease and/or response to treatment; or, for fatal conditions, a *post-mortem* examination. The gold standard could even be another laboratory test, with known validity, but which is too expensive or time-consuming for routine clinical use. Here, 'blind' refers to the fact that the gold-standard diagnosis should be made in ignorance of the test results. Similarly, the interpretation of the test results (are they positive or negative?) should be made without knowledge of the patients' true diagnostic state.

- Has the diagnostic test been evaluated in a sample that included patients with the appropriate range of severity of symptoms, treated and untreated patients, and those with commonly confused disorders? Was the sample drawn at random or through the use of subjective procedures? Was the population from which this sample is drawn similar to the one in which the diagnostic test is going to be used? Has the diagnostic test been independently evaluated by different investigators under a wide range of conditions?
- What are the reported estimates of the test's sensitivity and specificity? Do the authors provide the standard errors of these estimates (or, equivalently, do they provide the corresponding confidence intervals)? Are these small or unacceptably large? That is, was the sample size adequate for the job in hand?
- If you wished to replicate the evaluation of the test yourself, have the procedures been described in sufficient detail to permit an exact replication?
- If you decide to use a particular test or battery of tests, what are the benefits of being able to make a correct diagnosis? If a correct diagnosis makes no difference to prognosis, or decisions concerning treatment, then why bother? What are the potential costs of making mistakes?

2.6 USE OF MULTIPLE TESTS AND/OR SYMPTOMS

Now let us return to the overweight middle-aged man with chest pains. How would the results of two or more diagnostic tests be evaluated? The simple (but possible naïve) approach depends on the assumption that the diagnostic tests are all statistically independent. More subtle methods are beyond the scope of this text (see Strike, 1991, for example). Returning to the simple solution, statistical independence allows us to calculate a likelihood ratio for, say, three positive test results by forming the product of the three separate likelihoods as follows:

$$\textbf{Posterior odds} = \textbf{Prior odds} \times \textbf{LR(1)} \times \textbf{LR(2)} \times \textbf{LR(3)}$$

where LR(1), LR(2) and LR(3) are the likelihood ratios for tests 1, 2 and 3, respectively. If the tests are used in sequence we can keep adding test results until we can decide that the calculated posterior odds implies 'beyond reasonable doubt' (but not necessarily in the legal sense). Although the assumption of statistical independence is unlikely to hold in many situations, the multiplication of likelihood ratios has been found to work reasonably well in practice and has been widely employed in the development of diagnostic computer programs.

2.7 SUMMARY

This chapter has described the estimation and use of probabilities in the classification of patients to one of two or more mutually exclusive groups (diagnosis). The use of Bayes' theorem illustrates how one combines prior information with the results of a diagnostic test. Various problems of statistical inference have been described in the context of the estimation of a test's sensitivity and specificity. These are problems associated with the estimation of any unknown population characteristic (parameter) and they will be returned to in the later chapters. One aspect of a test's performance that has been ignored is that of its *reproducibility* or *precision*. Another is that of *diagnostic agreement* (or disagreement) amongst clinicians. Is the gold standard really 22 carat? These problems of *measurement* are the subject of the next chapter.

FURTHER READING

Inglefinger, J.A., Mosteller, F., Thibodeau, L.A. and Ware, J.H. (1983). *Biostatistics in clinical medicine* (Chapters 1 to 5). New York: Macmillan.

Jaeschke, R., Guyatt, G. and Sackett, D.L. (1994). Users' guides to the medical literature III. How to use an article about a diagnostic test A. Are the results of the study valid? *Journal of the American Medical Association* **271**, 389–91.

Jaeschke, R., Guyatt, G. and Sackett, D.L. (1994). Users' guides to the medical literature, III. How to use an article about a diagnostic test, B. What are the results and will they help me in caring for my patients? *Journal of the American Medical Association* **271**, 703–7.

Sackett, D.L., Haynes, R.B., Guyatt, G.H. and Tugwell, P. (1991). *Clinical Epidemiology* (2nd edition) (Chapters 1 to 5). Boston: Little, Brown.

EXERCISES

1 The prevalence of depression amongst GP attenders is about 30%. There are five people waiting in a doctor's waiting room. What is the probability that they are all depressed? What is the probability that none of them is depressed? What is the probability that at least one of them is depressed?

2 An investigator develops a screening test for cancer, and by using the test on *known* cancer and *known* non-cancer patients, determines that the test has a 2% false positive rate and a 12% false negative rate. In the population to which the test is to be applied it is assumed that 3% have undetected cancer. What are the sensitivity and specificity of the test? What is its likelihood ratio? Using Bayes' theorem, find the chance that someone with a positive test result actually has cancer.

3 Bland (1987) and Maxwell *et al.* (1983) discuss the possibility of using evidence of rib fractures as a method of detecting alcoholism. Among 74 patients with known alcoholic liver disease, 20 had evidence of at least one past fracture on chest X-ray. In a control group of 181 patients with non-alcoholic liver disease or gastrointestinal disorders only six had evidence of at least one fraction. What are the sensitivity, specificity and likelihood ratio of this 'test'? What are its positive predictive value and negative predictive value? Interpret your findings.

4 Assuming that a sample proportion (%) is distributed following the normal distribution, complete the following table:

Estimate of specificity (%)	Sample size	Standard error	95% C.I.	99% C.I.
25	10			
43	300			
76	50			
81	2000			
90	5000			
55	250			
68	30			
70	200			
79	1000			
85	100			

5 A patient with painful breast hardening is sent by her GP for mammography (a procedure for the study of the mammary gland by a specialized soft-tissue radiographic technique without injection of a radio-opaque contrast medium). The result is positive. Given the following information calculate the probability that the woman actually has breast cancer. (Key: M+ positive result on mammography; M− negative test result.)

P(Breast cancer in woman with painful breast hardening) = 0.01
P(M+ | no breast cancer)   = 0.1
P(M− | breast cancer)   = 0.1

The manipulation of probabilities also has uses other than assessing diagnostic test results. The following two exercises illustrate the use of elementary probability theory in genetics.

6 This example, taken from Elston and Johnson (1987), illustrates a situation that could arise in paternity testing (these days, however, it is more likely to involve DNA 'fingerprinting' than simple blood typing). Suppose a mother has blood type A (and hence genotype AA or AO), and her child's blood is type AB (and hence genotype AB). Thus the child's A gene came from the mother and the B gene must have come from the father. The mother alleges that a certain man is the father, and his blood is typed. The alleged father has blood type AB, and therefore genotype AB. What is required is the probability that the alleged father is in fact the true father. Make a number of simple assumptions and then apply Bayes' theorem to calculate the required probability.

7 Armitage and Berry (1987) illustrate the use of Bayes' theorem in genetic counselling. From genetic theory it is known that a woman with a haemophiliac brother has a probability of 0.5 of being a carrier of the disease. If she is, indeed, a carrier then there is also a probability of 0.5 that if she has a son he will have haemophilia. Suppose that she already has one son who does not have the illness. What is the (posterior) probability that the mother is a carrier? What is the probability that if she has a second son he too will be free of the illness?

The Variability of Clinical Measurements | 3

3.1 INTRODUCTION

Imagine that you are the middle-aged patient with chest pains referred to in the previous chapter. Your doctor has told you not to worry because she has decided that you are suffering from indigestion. She categorically rules out the risk of a heart attack. Despite this reassurance you may still be feeling a little anxious and may even decide to seek a second opinion. What is the probability that a second doctor, when presented with the same clinical evidence (or possibly after deciding to gather further evidence), will agree with the first one? Here you will clearly hope that the probability is quite high (i.e. close to 1), since indigestion, although unpleasant, is not life threatening. (If the first doctor had diagnosed a heart condition, you might be hoping for a rather lower probability of agreement!) Obviously we would like to believe that all doctors, faced with the same clinical evidence, will tend to agree with each other on a diagnosis. Anecdotes abound, however, that suggest that often they do not! In an ideal world the level of agreement would be perfect, but in the real one disagreements are bound to occur. In practice we would like to be able to estimate the extent of agreement (or disagreement) and take steps to minimize inconsistencies between doctors. Indices of agreement are the subject of Section 3.3.

Now suppose that, in coming to her diagnostic decision, your doctor has made use of a creatine kinase determination. Additionally, she is likely to have measured your blood pressure. In neither case will the measurement be infallible—it is bound to be subject to *measurement error*. If either of the measurements were to be repeated (by the same laboratory, in the case of the creatine kinase levels, or by the same doctor, in the case of blood pressure determination) then an identical result is unlikely to be obtained. There are bound to be fluctuations between replications of these measurements, but we hope that any changes will be small. If *different* laboratories were to carry out replicate determinations of creatine kinase concentrations there would again be fluctuations between the results which might, on average at least, be expected to be larger than when the same laboratory was involved. Similarly, fluctuations between blood pressure determinations made by *different* doctors are likely to be greater than those of repeated measurements made by the same doctor. The term **repeatability** is used to describe the variability of measurements made under near constant conditions (by the same laboratory using the same batch of reagents, for example), and **reproducibility** is used to describe the variability of measurements made under different conditions (by different laboratories or different doctors, for example).

There are often many sources of variability present at the same time. When a patient has his pulse rate measured by his doctor, its value will depend largely on some underlying 'true' value, characteristic of the patient. It will, however, also relate to the time of day that the measurement is made, whether the surgery is on the ground floor or up a flight of stairs, and whether or not the patient has smoked recently. Even characteristics regarded by many clinicians as essentially constant in healthy individuals, do vary. Body temperature, for example, where the long-held belief is that there is a 'normal value' of 98.4°F, has been shown to vary according to time of day, between 97.6°F in the early morning to a high of 98.5°F in the afternoon. Temperature also varies according to the sex of the individual, with women having slightly higher average temperatures than men.

The variability of measurement errors will be the subject of Section 3.4 but before discussing such detailed properties of measurements, it might be worthwhile to pause and consider what exactly is meant by the word 'measurement'. In the context of the present chapter, measurement is the process of allocating some sort of numerical value or label to an individual patient. An alternative term is **mensuration**.

You will no doubt be most familiar with the term measurement when used in the context of **quantitative** assessments (height, weight, blood pressure, etc). You may be less familiar with the idea of coding of a person's sex (1 = male; 2 = female), for example, as a form of measurement, or with treating a numerical code for a patient's diagnosis (1 = depression; 2 = anxiety; 3 = schizophrenia, etc.) as a measurement. For this reason, we start with a discussion of what we mean by the different *types* or *scales* of measurement.

3.2 TYPES OF MEASUREMENT

The basic material which forms the foundation of all medical investigations consists of the measurements and observations which are made on the individual patients being studied. Such measurement may, for example, involve determinations of blood pressure, weight and temperature. There may be an assessment of the pain being experienced by a patient, a statement about whether the patient is anxious or not, and often a record of how the patient's condition has improved after treatment, perhaps in terms of 'not improved,' 'slight improvement' and 'completely better.' Measurements taken in medical investigations are known collectively as *variables*, where a variable can be defined as any characteristic which may change in quantity or quality from one observation to the next.

Clearly not all measurement is the same. Measuring an individual's weight is qualitatively different from assessing their blood group. Measurement scales are differentiated essentially according to the degree of precision they can claim. If a clinician says that an individual has a high serum uric acid level, for example, it is not as precise as saying that the individual has 8.5 mg/100 ml of serum uric acid. The comment that a woman is tall is not as accurate as specifying that her height is 1.88 m. A useful classification of measurement scales is into *categorical (nominal)*, *ordinal*, *interval* and *ratio*.

Categorical or nominal measurements

The simplest type of observation on an individual is the allocation of that individual to one of several possible categories. A simple example is sex: male, female. Another example is marital status: single, married, divorced, widowed, other. The properties of such observations are:

- variable categories are *mutually exclusive*—an individual can

belong to only one category; and
- variable categories have **no logical order**—numbers may be assigned to categories but merely as convenient labels.

Ordinal measurements

When the categories of a nominal scale variable have some natural order an **ordinal scale measurement** results. A psychiatrist, for example, may grade patients in terms of their perceived anxiety as 'not anxious', 'mildly anxious', 'moderately anxious' or 'severely anxious', and use the numbers 0, 1, 2 and 3 to label the categories; here *lower* numbers indicate *less* anxiety. Consequently the numbers representing the anxiety categories of a sample of patients would allow the psychiatrist to arrange the patients in order of their degree of anxiety from lowest to highest. In other words, it would be possible to **rank** the patients with respect to their anxiety level. The numbers assigned to the anxiety categories would not, however, allow the psychiatrist to say anything about the *differences* in anxiety of patients. With measurements on an ordinal scale, a difference of say a single point on the scale at different parts of the scale, does not necessarily represent equal differences in anxiety. In other words, the difference in anxiety between patients with a 'mildly anxious' (1) and 'moderately anxious' (2) rating is not necessarily the same as that between patients assigned categories 'not anxious' (0) and 'mildly anxious' (1). The numbers used to label the categories usually only have **rank order** significance.

The following are the properties of an ordinal scale:

- variable categories are **mutually exclusive**,
- variable categories have some **logical order**, and
- variable categories are scaled according to the **amount or intensity** of the particular characteristic they possess.

Interval and ratio scales of measurement

Measurements on an interval scale possess all the properties of an ordinal scale plus the additional feature that equal differences on any part of the scale are equivalent. Consider, for example, temperature on the Fahrenheit scale. The difference in temperature of two patients with values of 98.6°F and 100°F is the same as that between patients with temperatures of 97°F and 98.4°F. Note, however, that the zero point on the Fahrenheit scale of temperature is simply another point on the scale; it does *not* represent the complete absence of heat (lower temperatures are indicated by negative values). Neither is an object with a temperature of 100°F twice as hot as one with temperature 50°F. Degrees Fahrenheit is an interval but not a *ratio* scale. To qualify as the latter a scale must have a zero point which represents the complete absence of the characteristic being measured. Height and weight are obvious ratio scale measurements, so that a person of 200lbs *can* be said to be twice as heavy as another person weighing only 100lbs. Temperature measured in degrees Kelvin *is* a ratio scale since the zero point on this scale (absolute zero), corresponds to a complete lack of molecular motion and hence absence of heat. Consequently a temperature of 50°K does represent twice the warmth of 25°K.

Interval and ratio scales are often *continuous* measurements. Temperature, for example, could in principle take any value on a continuum, although the accuracy of the measuring instrument will restrict its measurement to some particular number of decimal places. But some interval scales, by definition, can only have *discrete* or *integral* values. Examples include the number of symptoms of depression, the number of prior episodes of a recurring illness, the number of children in a family, and so on.

In the following sections we will discuss the variability of just two types of measurement: firstly, a nominal measure—diagnosis (presence/absence of a particular disease); secondly, (strictly speaking an ordinal measure), but one which will be treated as if it were interval—a measure of psychological distress obtained by administering the General Health Questionnaire (Goldberg, 1972). These two examples have been chosen to give you an insight into the problems involved in determining the consistency of replicated measurements. There would be little point in cataloguing all the possible statistical approaches for all the possible types of measurement scale. (Such details can, if required, be found in Dunn, 1989.)

3.3 DIAGNOSTIC AGREEMENT

Here we are concerned with agreement (or disagreement) between categorical or nominal measurements. To simplify the discussion we will look at a straightforward example involving a judgement concerning the presence or absence of a particular characteristic. A doctor, for example, might simply record whether or not she considers that a patient is suffering from depression. A hypothetical example involving the judgements of *two* doctors for the same 29 patients is given in Display 3.1. A summary of these data, in the form of what is known as a **contingency table**, is provided in Display 3.2. There are a total of 22 agreements (75.9%)—10 patients on which the two clinicians agree about the absence of depression, and 12 on which they agree about its presence. There are seven patients (24.1%) who receive a diagnosis of depression from Doctor A but not from Doctor B. These are the disagreements. There are no patients who receive a diagnosis of depression from Doctor B but not from Doctor A. It appears that the probability of Doctor A diagnosing depression (65.5%) might be higher than that for Doctor B (41.4%), but to what extent do the two doctors agree in their diagnoses of depression?

The most intuitively obvious index of agreement for the observations in Display 3.2 is simply the proportion of agreements between the two doctors, $22/29 = 0.76$. But although this index does have the virtue of simplicity, it ignores a possibly important component of the diagnostic exercise, namely the agreement between the two doctors that would be obtained if they were simply applying the labels 'depressed' and 'not depressed' to patients at random in accordance with their particular **marginal rates**, 65.5% and 34.5% for Doctor A, and 41.4% and 58.6% for Doctor B. An index that corrects for this **chance agreement** is the **kappa coefficient**.

Remembering the multiplication rule for probabilities (Section 2.2), the expected chance agreement for saying 'no depression' is $58.6 \times 34.5 = 20.2\%$. Similarly, the chance-expected agreement for saying 'depression' is $41.4 \times 65.5 = 27.2\%$. The overall agreement expected by chance is therefore simply the total of these two values, that is, 47.4%. The agreement observed, over and above that expected by chance, is therefore $75.9 - 47.4 = 28.5\%$. The maximum possible improvement would have been $100.0 - 47.4 = 52.6\%$. The kappa coefficient is simply the ratio, $28.5/52.6 = 0.54$.

In summary,

$$\text{Kappa} = \frac{\text{Observed agreement} - \text{Chance agreement}}{\text{Maximum possible agreement} - \text{Chance agreement}}$$

leading to, in our example

Hypothetical data on 29 patients			
Patient	Doctor A	Doctor B	Agreement
1	no	yes	no
2	no	no	yes
3	no	no	yes
4	yes	yes	yes
5	no	no	yes
6	yes	yes	yes
7	no	no	yes
8	no	no	yes
9	no	no	yes
10	yes	yes	yes
11	no	yes	no
12	yes	yes	yes
13	no	no	yes
14	yes	yes	yes
15	yes	yes	yes
16	no	yes	no
17	no	yes	no
18	no	yes	no
19	yes	yes	yes
20	no	no	yes
21	yes	yes	yes
22	yes	yes	yes
23	no	no	yes
24	no	no	yes
25	yes	yes	yes
26	no	yes	no
27	no	yes	no
28	yes	yes	yes
29	yes	yes	yes
Number of yes ratings:	12	19	
Number of agreements:			22

DISPLAY 3.1 Agreement between two doctors on the diagnosis of depression

$$\text{Kappa} = \frac{75.9 - 47.4}{100.0 - 47.4} = 0.54$$

An alternative (and equivalent) way of expressing kappa is the following:

Counts (% in brackets)		Doctor A		
		No	Yes	Total
Doctor B	No	10 (34.5)	7 (24.1)	17 (58.6)
	Yes	0 (0.0)	12 (41.4)	12 (41.4)
	Totals	10 (34.5)	19 (65.5)	29

DISPLAY 3.2 Summary of the data from Display 3.1

$$\text{Kappa} = 1 - \frac{\text{Observed disagreement}}{\text{Disagreement expected by chance}}$$

$$= 1 - \frac{24.1}{52.6}$$

$$= 0.54, \text{ as before.}$$

Both the observed and chance-expected percentage of disagreements are simply 100 minus the corresponding percentage of agreements. The reason for introducing this alternative expression for kappa is because it has a similar form to the measure of reliability to be described in Section 3.4.

Although it is theoretically possible to obtain a negative value for kappa, in practice values are observed that range from zero (no agreement above chance) to unity (perfect agreement). What about the value of 0.54? Is this an indication of good agreement? This is a difficult question to answer. There are no objective criteria by which to judge kappa coefficients. Perhaps a better question might be 'Does the kappa coefficient indicate that agreement is good enough?', but again this would depend on subjective judgement. A rough guide is provided by Display 3.3, but this should not be taken too seriously.

Clearly the above kappa of 0.54 is also estimated from a fairly small sample of patients. If the exercise were to be repeated for further samples of 29 patients there would be considerable sampling variation in the values of kappa obtained.

What is the standard error of the kappa coefficient? The required formula is rather complicated and is provided in Display 3.4. The

Kappa	Strength of agreement
0.01	poor
0.01–0.20	slight
0.21–0.40	fair
0.41–0.60	moderate
0.61–0.80	substantial
0.81–1.00	almost perfect

DISPLAY 3.3 What is good agreement? (from Landis and Koch, 1977)

use of this formula on our data leads to a value for se(κ) of 0.14. An approximate 95% confidence interval for a kappa coefficient is obtained by taking the observed kappa value ± 1.96 standard errors. For the present example this leads to the interval (0.26, 0.82). So in terms of the statements in Display 3.3, agreement here is somewhere between fair and almost perfect.

3.4 REPEATABILITY AND RELIABILITY OF QUANTITATIVE MEASUREMENTS

Display 3.5 shows data arising from a small study in which twelve clinical psychology students were asked to complete the 12-item version of the General Health Questionnaire (GHQ) (Goldberg, 1972) on one day, and then again three days later. This is an example of what a psychologist might call a *test–retest reliability study*. A high GHQ score indicates psychological distress (anxiety and depression, for example); a low score is indicative of a lack of problems. Each item has four possible graded responses, here coded as 0, 1, 2 or 3, and to produce the total GHQ score the 12-item responses are simply added together. The total score can therefore range from 0 to 36.

First, consider ways in which the data as a whole might be summarized. What is a typical or average value (sometimes called a *measure of location*)? The most commonly used measure is the *arithmetic mean* (the sum of all the scores divided by the number of observations). For the GHQ data the mean is 10.17. Next an index of the variability (*dispersion*) of the data is required. One possibility would be to use the *range* of the observations, i.e. the difference

Consider the following observed proportions, where N is the total number of patients judged by two doctors, A and B:

		Doctor A		
		No	Yes	Total (marginal proportion)
Doctor B	No	p_{11}	p_{12}	p_{1+}
	Yes	p_{21}	p_{22}	p_{2+}
	Total	p_{+1}	p_{+2}	1

Let $P_o = (p_{11} + p_{22})$ be the observed agreement (measured as a proportion) and $P_c = (p_{1+}p_{+1} + p_{2+}p_{+2})$ be the corresponding chance value. Then kappa (κ) is given by the expression

$$\kappa = (P_o - P_c)/(1 - P_c)$$

and its sampling variance is

$$var(\kappa) = \frac{\{A + B + C\}}{N(1 - P_c)^4}$$

where

$A = p_{11}[(1 - P_c) - (p_{+1} + p_{1+})(1 - P_o)]^2 + p_{22}[(1 - P_c) - (p_{+2} + p_{2+})(1 - P_o)]^2$

$B = (1 - P_o)^2 [p_{12}(p_{+1} + p_{2+})^2 + p_{21}(p_{+2} + p_{1+})^2]$

and

$C = (P_o P_c - 2P_c + P_o)^2$

The standard error of κ, se(κ), is simply(!) the square root of var(κ).

DISPLAY 3.4 Calculation of the sandard error of kappa (for a binary yes/no judgement)

between the largest and smallest values, giving here the values $24 - 2 = 22$. Although the range is very simple to calculate it is not a good measure of variability; it uses only a very small amount of the information in the data (just two values) and may be very badly distorted by the presence of **outliers** (see Section 3.6).

More satisfactory measures of dispersion are the sample **variance** and the sample **standard deviation**. (These two measures are, essentially, equivalent, since the standard deviation is the square

Subject	1st GHQ score	2nd GHQ score	Difference	Squared difference
1	12	12	0	0
2	8	7	−1	1
3	22	24	−2	4
4	10	14	−4	16
5	10	8	2	4
6	6	4	2	4
7	8	5	3	9
8	4	6	−2	4
9	14	14	0	0
10	6	5	1	1
11	2	5	−3	9
12	22	16	6	36
			Sum:	88
			Mean:	7.33

DISPLAY 3.5 Test-retest results for GHQ scores (from Dunn, 1992)

root of the variance. The former gives an index of variability in the same units as the original measurements.) The variance is basically the arithmetic mean of the squared deviations of each of the 24 observations from their overall mean (except that, for technical reasons beyond the scope of this text, one obtains the mean squared deviation by dividing their sum by the sample size *minus one* instead of the sample size itself). The calculations are illustrated in Display 3.6. The variance of the GHQ scores is 37.19 and, therefore, their standard deviation is 6.10 (the square root of 37.19). The overall variance can be thought of as a measure of the variability of (or disagreement between) the observations when the matching of test and retest scores is ignored. In the context of the last section on agreement, it is equivalent to a measure of chance–expected disagreement for randomly paired observations.

Returning to the main aim of the analysis, the investigation of the disagreements between the observed test and retest GHQ scores, we can determine the mean of the differences (score at time 1 minus score at time 2). This is 0.17. This is relatively small and there appears to be little evidence of a systematic change in GHQ scores over the three days between the first and second tests. If we are

Subject	Time	GHQ score	Deviation from mean*	Squared deviation
1	1	12	1.83	3.36
1	2	12	1.83	3.36
2	1	8	−2.17	4.69
2	2	7	−3.17	10.03
3	1	22	11.83	140.03
3	2	24	13.83	191.36
4	1	10	−0.17	0.03
4	2	14	3.83	14.69
5	1	10	−0.17	0.03
5	2	8	−2.17	4.69
6	1	6	−4.17	17.36
6	2	4	−6.17	38.03
7	1	8	−2.17	4.69
7	2	5	−5.17	26.69
8	1	4	−6.17	38.03
8	2	6	−4.17	17.36
9	1	14	3.83	14.69
9	2	14	3.83	14.69
10	1	6	−4.17	17.36
10	2	5	−5.17	26.69
11	1	2	−8.17	66.69
11	2	5	−5.17	26.69
12	1	22	11.83	140.03
12	2	16	5.83	34.03

Total: 855.00

*GHQ score minus the mean GHQ score (10.1667)

Variance = 855/23
= 37.19
S.D. = sqrt (37.19)
= 6.10

DISPLAY 3.6 Calculation of the variance and standard deviation for the GHQ scores in Display 3.5

prepared to assume that the difference between test and retest scores only arises from independent random measurement errors then we can estimate the variance of the individual measurement errors from the mean of the squared differences divided by two. That is, from Display 3.5:

$$\text{Mean squared difference} = 88/12$$

$$= 7.33$$

$$\text{Variance of errors} = 7.33/2$$

$$= 3.67$$

Therefore,

$$\text{S.D. of errors} = 1.91$$

In psychology the standard deviation of the measurement errors is called the **standard error of measurement** (do not confuse this with the standard error of a mean, to be introduced later). The standard error of measurement is a measure of repeatability of the measurement. Equivalently, the standard error of measurement is a measure of the precision of a test instrument: the lower the standard error of measurement the higher the test's precision. The higher the test's precision the more confident we can be that a subject's true or error-free score is close to that actually observed. In fact, we can calculate a 95% confidence interval for an individual's test score by assuming that measurement errors are normally distributed about a mean of zero. We simply then take the observed score ± 1.96 standard errors of measurement. The standard error of measurement would, of course, have to be known fairly precisely—from a large data set—not from a small sample of 12 subjects!

An index of agreement or **reliability** (R) can be calculated from the variance of the errors (3.67) and the overall variance (37.19) in an analogous manner to the calculation of a kappa coefficient, as follows:

$$\textbf{R} = \textbf{1} - \frac{\textbf{Observed disagreement}}{\textbf{Chance–expected disagreement}}$$

$$= 1 - 3.67/37.19$$

$$= 0.90$$

R will vary from zero (no reliability) to unity (perfect reliability). It is a measure of how well a particular test or measurement can distinguish individuals within a given population. The ratio 3.67/37.19 is the proportion of the variation explained by measurement error. It follows that R is the proportion of the variation that is *not* due to measurement error. That is, it is the proportion in the variability of the measurements that is explained by variation in the subjects being measured. Another interpretation of reliability will be given in the next section.

If we know a test's reliability (from consulting the test's manual, for example, or by calculating it as in the following section) and the overall standard deviation (S.D.) of the test scores, we can re-arrange the above formula for R to provide the test's standard error of measurement (S.E.M.):

$$S.E.M. = S.D. \times sqrt(1 - R)$$

If, for example, we know that $R = 0.95$ and S.D. $= 15$, then

$$S.E.M. = 15 \times sqrt(1 - 0.95)$$
$$= 3.35$$

Before leaving this section, perhaps it would be useful to add a note of caution. The reliability coefficient is characteristic *both* of the subjects being measured *and* of the quality of the measuring device being assessed. For a fixed standard error of measurement (repeatability), variation in the heterogeneity of the subjects (as measured by their standard deviation, S.D.) will change the value of R. An increase in the S.D. will increase R; a decrease will decrease R. The reliability of a test or other measuring device is not a measure of its precision (that is the role of repeatability), but is a measure of how well it will discriminate between subjects in a given population (that is, with a given standard deviation). Similarly, a kappa coefficient for agreement on the presence or absence of a particular disease, for example, is also dependent on the prevalence of the disease (i.e. the proportion of the subjects with the disease) in the population. It, too, is population-dependent.

3.5 AN INTRODUCTION TO CORRELATION

Before developing the discussion on the reliability of measurements, let us digress for a moment to look at a different clinical problem. Suppose a clinician working in a small hospital in Scotland wishes to investigate whether or not there is any relationship between mater-nal alcohol consumption during pregnancy and a baby's resulting birth weight; in particular, whether excessive drinking during preg-nancy has a tendency to result in a child with a low birth weight.

Clearly the investigator cannot study all pregnant women (on Earth, in the United Kingdom or even in Scotland!). In fact it is likely that she will only be able to study the pregnant women attending her own hospital during a particular period, say, of one year. It is from this *sample* of pregnant women that she will collect information on drinking habits and record the weight of each woman's baby. One of her tasks will then be to describe and summarize the observations, *particularly* the observed association between maternal drinking and the baby's birth weight. Imagine that she has studied a sample of 100 women, collected information about the amount of alcohol consumed during pregnancy, and weighed their babies. She now wishes to describe and interpret what she has found. Summarizing and quantifying the relationships between pairs of variables is an extremely important part of many medical investigations, and generally involves the use of the *scatter plot* (*scatter diagram*, *scattergram*) and calculation of a *correlation coefficient*.

The scatter plot (or scatter diagram)

The scatter plot is simply an x, y plot, with the x values being the observations on one of the two variables and the y values being the observations on the other. Such a diagram for the birth weight and alcohol consumption data is shown in Display 3.7. Here there is certainly no very obvious relationship between the two variables, although there is perhaps a slight tendency for low birth weights to be associated with high alcohol consumption. Display 3.8 shows the relationship between the first and second GHQ scores listed in Display 3.5. Here there is evidence of a strong relationship—as one would hope that there would be considering that they are supposedly both measures of the same thing!

The correlation coefficient

Although the scatter plot is an extremely useful (and essential) first step in assessing the relationship between two variables, it generally needs to be supplemented by calculating a statistic known as the *correlation coefficient*, usually denoted by r. This coefficient quantifies both the *direction* and the *strength* of the observed relationship. This allows easy comparison of the relationships of different pairs of variables. For the alcohol consumption–birth-weight data r is -0.19; the correlation between first and second GHQ scores is 0.90. The

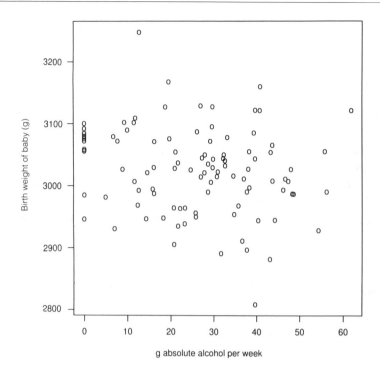

DISPLAY 3.7 Plot of children's birth weights against amounts of maternal drinking during pregnancy

correlation coefficient is calculated from the observed pairs of values as shown in Display 3.9 (using the GHQ data as an example). First we estimate the mean of the two variables and then determine the deviations of each of the individual observations from their respective means (as in the case of calculation of the sample variance). If two variables are positively associated then a large positive deviation for one of them will tend to be matched by a positive one on the other. Similarly, negative deviations will also appear together. In both situations the product of the two deviations will be positive. If, on the other hand, the two variables are negatively associated, one of the variables will tend to have a positive deviation when the other's is negative, and vice versa. In this case the product of the deviations will tend to be negative.

The *covariance* of two variables is basically the average of the products of the above deviations from the variables' means (but again the sum of products is divided by $N - 1$, where N is the sample size, as in the case of the variance). The corresponding correlation

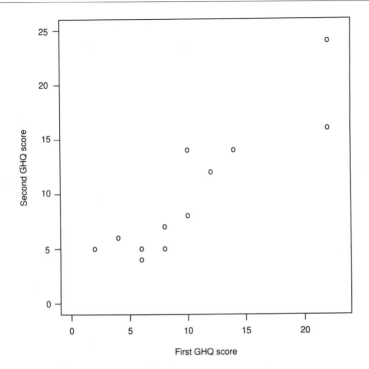

DISPLAY 3.8 Plot of second GHQ score against the first GHQ score (using data from Display 3.5)

coefficient is the covariance divided by the product of the variables' standard deviations (equivalent to the sum of products divided by the square root of the product of the two sums of squared deviations). Remembering the formula for calculating the correlation coefficient, r, is not of great importance, it *is* essential to understand how to interpret such coefficients and, in addition, to understand under what circumstances they can be misleading. With this in mind, Display 3.10 shows a number of scatter plots and the associated values of r. Firstly the *sign* of r indicates the direction of the relationship between the two variables, and the *numerical value* of r, the strength of the relationship. A positive correlation indicates that the two variables tend to be large together or small together, whereas as a negative sign implies that one variable takes large values when the other is small and vice versa. If the values lie exactly on a straight line (excluding one which is horizontal), the correlation coefficient takes either the value $+1$, or -1, depending on the direction of the line. The correlation coefficient cannot exceed $+1$, or be less than -1. One other rather special value of the correlation coefficient is zero. This implies that there is no *linear* relationship between the two variables (see below).

Essentially, r is a measure of the scatter of the points in the scatter plot around an underlying linear trend (straight line); the greater the spread of the points above and below the line, the lower the correlation. One way of assessing the importance of a particular value of r is to square it; r^2 is the proportion of the variability of one of the two measures which is explained by the variation in the other (again, assuming that the relationship is linear). An r of 0.5 between variables x and y, for example, indicates that 25% of the variability of y is explained by variation in x (and vice versa). A correlation of -0.90 is equivalent to 81%, 0.4 to 16%, and so on. For most practical purposes a correlation of 0.4 or less (ignoring the sign) is unlikely to be of great **clinical significance**.

If the relationship between the two variables is other than linear, then r is not an appropriate summary of the relationship and could

Subject	1st GHQ	2nd GHQ	Deviation of 1st GHQ from its mean	Deviation of 2nd GHQ from its mean	Product of deviations
1	12	12	1.67	2.00	3.34
2	8	7	−2.33	−3.00	6.99
3	22	24	11.67	14.00	163.38
4	10	14	−0.33	4.00	−1.32
5	10	8	−0.33	−2.00	0.66
6	6	4	−4.33	−6.00	25.98
7	8	5	−2.33	−5.00	11.65
8	4	6	−6.33	−4.00	25.32
9	14	14	3.67	4.00	14.68
10	6	5	−4.33	−5.00	21.65
11	2	5	−8.33	−5.00	41.65
12	22	16	11.67	6.00	70.02
Mean:	10.33	10.00			

Sum of squared deviations: 446.666   408.000
Sum of products of deviations: 384.000
Correlation coefficient (r): 384/sqrt(446.666 × 408.000)
          = 0.90

DISPLAY 3.9 Illustrative calculations for a correlation (using the GHQ data from Display 3.5)

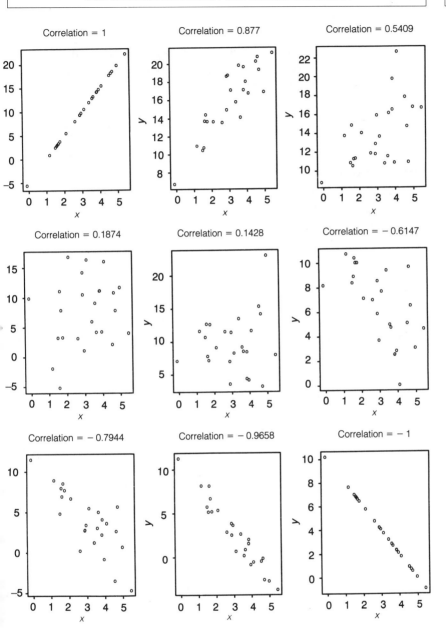

DISPLAY 3.10 Illustrative scatter plots

take the value zero (or some value very close to zero) even when the two variables were strongly related. Display 3.11 shows an example. One further point about the correlation coefficient is that its value can be heavily influenced by the presence of outlying observations (see next section).

The value of r calculated from a sample of N pairs of variable values can be used to provide a confidence interval for the population correlation although the details, given in Display 3.12, are a little involved. For the maternal alcohol/baby's birth weight example the 95% confidence interval is $(-0.37, 0.01)$. Note that this includes the value zero so it is quite possible that there is *no* linear association between the two variables in the population although a small negative value is perhaps more likely.

Intra-class correlation

Now let us return to another aspect of the reliability of clinical measurements and suppose that the repeated GHQ scores given in Display 3.5 were just replicate measurements, as would often be the

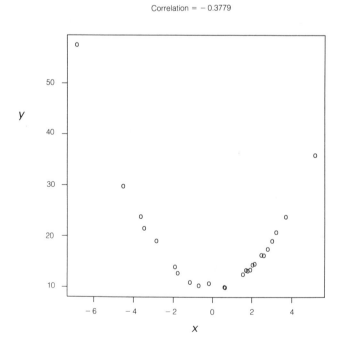

Correlation = − 0.3779

DISPLAY 3.11 Scatter plot for a non-linear relationship

(a) The formulae

Let the estimated correlation be r, based on a sample of size N. Fisher's z transformation is given by

$$z = 0.5 \times [\log_e(1+r) - \log_e(1-r)]$$
$$= 0.5 \times \log_e[(1+r)/(1-r)]$$

Fisher's z is a Normally distributed random variable with a standard error, se(z), equal to $1/\text{sqrt}(N-3)$. Consequently a 95% CI for z has the limits

$$z - 1.96 \times \text{se}(z) \text{ to } z + 1.96 \times \text{se}(z)$$

To obtain the corresponding limits for z itself, we apply the following inverse transformation:

$$r = (e^{2z} - 1)/(e^{2z} + 1)$$

where z is replaced in the above calculation by its upper and lower confidence limits in turn. (It is more usual to use statistical tables to look up the required value of z for a given estimate of correlation, and also to obtain the upper and lower limits for r after calculation of the corresponding values for z.)

(b) Example using the GHQ data

$$r = 0.90 \ (N = 12)$$
$$z = 0.5 \times \log_e[(1+0.9)/(1-0.9)]$$
$$= 1.472$$
$$\text{se}(z) = 1/3$$
$$= 0.333$$

95% CI for z is given by

lower limit: $1.472 - 1.96 \times 0.333 = 0.8193$
upper limit: $1.472 + 1.96 \times 0.333 = 2.1247$

Therefore, lower limit for r is

$$(e^{2 \times 0.8193} - 1)/(e^{2 \times 0.8193} + 1) = 0.67$$

The corresponding upper limit for r is

$$(e^{2 \times 2.1247} - 1)/(e^{2 \times 2.1247} + 1) = 0.97$$

DISPLAY 3.12 Calculation of 95% confidence interval (CI) for a correlation coefficient: Fisher's transformation

case with biochemical or physical measures. That is, there is no element of time involved—one could present the pairs of observations in any order without affecting the interpretation of the data. In this case it is difficult to calculate a correlation coefficient as in Display 3.9. This problem is solved, however, by calculation of an *intra-class correlation*. This is achieved by entering each pair of observations twice, once in each of the two possible orders, into a 'double' table as in Display 3.13. The calculation then proceeds as in the calculation of the *product-moment correlation* (the full name for the correlation coefficient whose calculation is illustrated in Display 3.9).

Display 3.13 illustrates the calculations involved. In the case of the GHQ scores the product-moment and intra-class correlations happen to be almost identical, but this is not necessarily the case. Usually the intra-class correlation will be the smaller (closer to zero) of the two correlations. In general, too, it will be a better estimate of reliability (agreement) as described in Section 3.4; the product-moment correlation is more appropriately thought of as a *measure of association*. Two perfectly calibrated thermometers, one scaled in degrees Centigrade, and the other Fahrenheit, will show perfect association (the product-moment correlation will equal 1), but nothing like perfect agreement (i.e. they will provide an intra-class correlation less than 1). In fact, it might not make a lot of sense to talk about agreement between instruments known to be calibrated in different ways. Returning to the Scottish doctor, it would be senseless for her to talk about the agreement between measures of mothers' alcohol consumption and their babies' birth weights!

A confidence interval for an intra-class correlation can be determined in exactly the same way as for the product-moment correlation, but remember to base the calculation of the standard errors using N, the number of independent pairs of observations, and not $2N$, as might be inferred mistakenly by use of the 'doubled' table.

3.6 THE INFLUENCE OF OUTLYING OBSERVATIONS

One of the problems arising in any statistical analysis is the fact that the results and conclusions can often be distorted by one or two influential observations. Most commonly, we might have one or two very unusual measurements which might arise from the fact that we are investigating a very unusual subject or patient. Often, however,

Subject	GHQ scores		Deviations from overall mean		Product of deviations
1	12	12	1.83	1.83	3.36
1	12	12	1.83	1.83	3.36
2	8	7	−2.17	−3.17	6.86
2	7	8	−3.17	−2.17	6.86
3	22	24	11.83	13.83	163.69
3	24	22	13.83	11.83	163.69
4	10	14	−0.17	3.83	−0.64
4	14	10	3.83	−0.17	−0.64
5	10	8	−0.17	−2.17	0.36
5	8	10	−2.17	−0.17	0.36
6	6	4	−4.17	−6.17	25.69
6	4	6	−6.17	−4.17	25.69
7	8	5	−2.17	−5.17	11.19
7	5	8	−5.17	−2.17	11.19
8	4	6	−6.17	−4.17	25.69
8	6	4	−4.17	−6.17	25.69
9	14	14	3.83	3.83	14.69
9	14	14	3.83	3.83	14.69
10	6	5	−4.17	−5.17	21.53
10	5	6	−5.17	−4.17	21.53
11	2	5	−8.17	−5.17	42.19
11	5	2	−5.17	−8.17	42.19
12	22	16	11.83	5.83	69.03
12	16	22	5.83	11.83	69.03

Mean: 10.17
Sum of squared deviations: 855.36
Sum of products of deviations: 767.28
Intra-class correlation: 767.28/855.36
=0.90

DISPLAY 3.13 Calculations for an intra-class correlation (using 'double' table)

we have simply made a mistake either in taking an instrument reading or in subsequently transferring the information to a computer (or, if we are a badly organized worker, in transcribing it from a scrap of paper to a laboratory notebook). Whatever the cause of these unusual observations (termed *statistical outliers*) it is important that we be aware of their possible influence and check for their presence.

First, let us consider the influence of outliers on means and variances (and, by implication, on standard deviations, reliabilities and correlation coefficients). Returning to the GHQ scores in Display 3.5, suppose that we had carelessly entered the value 66 for the first GHQ score of subject 6 (actual GHQ score = 6). Now, you might think that it would be obvious to anyone that this is a mistake. It is not even in the permitted range (from 0 to 36). But, unfortunately, it is very easy to miss errors such as these, and they very often are missed—particularly when the set of data is much larger than this one. Having failed to see our mistake, we calculate the overall mean and variance of all of the 24 GHQ scores as in Section 3.4. We obtain a mean of 12.67 and a variance of 165.45 (corresponding to the original values of 10.17 and 37.19, respectively). Inevitably they have both changed as a result of our mistake. The mean, in this example, has not shifted too far, but the impact on the sample variance is enormous! Now, if we look at the difference between first and second GHQ scores, we obtain a mean of 5.33 and a variance of 326.06 (corresponding to the original values of 0.17 and 7.97, respectively). They have both now changed quite dramatically. Half of the mean of the squared differences is $327.33/2 = 163.67$, giving a new standard error of measurement of 12.79 (originally it was 1.91) and the new estimate of reliability, estimated by $1 - 163.67/165.45$, is, for all practical purposes, zero. The correlation between first and second GHQ scores is 0.02!

The above summary statistics (mean, variance, standard deviation and the various correlation or reliability coefficients) are all influenced by outliers, and often dramatically so. They are described as being **sensitive** to the presence of outliers. This implies that the detection of outliers is an extremely important part of any statistical analysis. How do we do it? First, we make plots and other graphical displays. These are discussed in more detail in the following chapter, but here, for example, a scatter plot for the first GHQ score plotted against the second GHQ score (see Display 3.14) clearly reveals our error. This example illustrates how vital it is to examine the corresponding scatter plots when estimating correlations (reliabilities) between variables. Knowing the permitted range of our GHQ scores, we should have also looked at the observed range to make sure that nothing fell outside that permitted. The range of the observed differences (-4 to $+64$) should also have aroused our suspicions!

Apart from detecting outlying observations and, if appropriate,

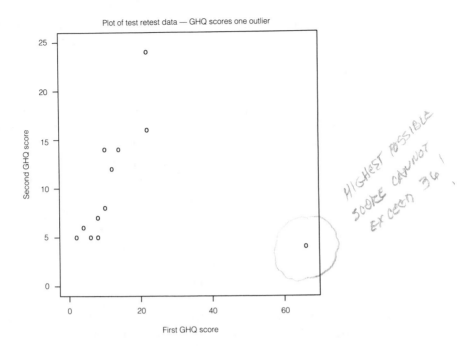

DISPLAY 3.14 Scatter plot with outlier

removing them, an alternative strategy is to use summary statistics that are *not* sensitive to their influences—that is, to use statistics that are **outlier-resistant**. A commonly used example of a resistant measure of location (typical value), for example, is the **median**. To determine the median we put all the observations in rank order (from the smallest to the largest, or vice versa) and then select the middle value. The median is the value that splits the sample in half; that is, half of the subjects have observations less than the median, and half have values which have more. The median is the middle value for an odd number of observations, or the mean of the two middle values for an even number. For the 24 GHQ scores in Display 3.5 the median is 8.00. If the observations were distributed symmetrically around a central value then one would expect the median and mean to be about the same (the mean in this case was 10.17). The fact that the median is smaller than the mean indicates **positive skewness**—there are relatively more low values than one would expect of a symmetrical distribution and a few quite large ones. This is one of the characteristics of the GHQ score when used on samples of non-patients: most of the people do not have many problems, but a few do. One would expect the differences between first and second GHQ scores, on the other hand, to be more or less symmetrically distributed. The median difference is 0.00 (compared to the mean of 0.17).

Now let us introduce the outlier (66) as before. The median of the GHQ scores is 9.00, and that for the differences is 0.50. The outlier has had hardly any impact in either case. This is what we mean by outlier-resistant. Now consider a resistant measure of variability. One possibility is the *inter-quartile range* (IQR)—this is the range across the middle half of the data (that is, the range of values remaining after the smallest 25% and the largest 25% of the values have been temporarily discarded). To determine the IQR we take the rank ordered values, determine the lower quartile (the value which divides the sample into a lower quarter and an upper three-quarters) and also the upper quartile (the value which divides the sample into a lower three-quarters and an upper quarter). The difference in the values of the lower and upper quartiles is the IQR. The IQR for the GHQ scores in Display 3.5 is equal to 8.75. The IQR for the differences is 4.00. If we introduce the outlier (66) these values remain at 8.75 and 4.00. There has been no change at all! Although this will not always be the case, we would, in general, expect that outliers would have very little influence on an inter-quartile range.

How do we use these summary statistics in practice? We usually wish to work with sensitive summary statistics to estimate reliabilities and repeatabilities (standard errors of measurement). We also tend to use the sensitive statistics such as means and variances (or, equivalently, standard deviations) in many statistical tests and in the construction of confidence intervals. If this is so then our data will need to be very carefully checked for outliers through the use of plots and summary statistics. If we calculate both resistant and sensitive summary statistics and then find that they are very similar (the mean is more-or-less equal to the median, and the standard deviation is, very roughly, half the IQR) then we have little to worry about. If they are very different we have a problem and we have to identify its source (one or more outliers, for example) and decide how to eliminate it. We may decide that we need to transform the original measurements (by taking logarithms, for example) to make them more symmetrical or, if we can convince ourselves that the outliers are blunders, either eliminate the outlying observations or correct them (the latter being preferable).

3.7 CRITICAL APPRAISAL OF PUBLISHED RELIABILITY STUDIES

The questions to be asked by readers of reliability or precision studies are very similar to those asked in the corresponding section of Chapter 2 (Section 2.5). We will assume, however, that it might be useful to go over the same points again, but from a slightly different perspective.

- Have there been truly independent ratings or measurements made on each of the patients or specimens? Are the assessments really blind? Can we really assume, for example, that subjects cannot remember what responses they gave to a questionnaire filled in three days previously (see Display 3.5)? When an investigator takes replicate test readings is he or she likely to repeat the same error on both occasions? Many biochemical tests illustrate random matrix effects (specimen by assay method interactions). What is meant by this? Specimens contain bio-chemical components other than the one being assayed and some of them will interfere with the assay. A given specimen will cause a given amount of interference (that is, the amount of interference being characteristic of each specimen) which will remain constant across replications of the assay for this partic-ular specimen.

  Another source of lack of independence arises in studies of rater agreement, when the ratings are supposedly independently determined by each of the members of a panel of clinicians after they have watched a clinical interview given by another clinician through a half-silvered mirror, or have watched a video-tape or listened to an audio-tape of the same interview. Even allowing for the fact that this design cannot investigate sources of variation due to interviewer effects (with the possibility of different interviews eliciting different information), there are likely to be several additional reasons why members of the panel might come to more similar conclusions than might be the case if they had each investigated the patient's symptoms completely independently. They are likely to be influenced by pauses, non-verbal reactions and other clues hinting at what the interviewing clinician might be thinking (as well as the order in which the questions are asked).

- Have the measurements been made on a representative sample of patients or specimens? In particular, is it clear that the investigators have not discarded difficult cases from the study? In terms of your own potential use of the measurement procedure, is the population which you intend to use it on comparable to the one the investigators sampled from? If not, what effect is this likely to have on a kappa or reliability coefficient, for example? Perhaps you should always check what is likely to happen by always checking the reliability of your own assessments and measurements. One would, of course, expect clinical chemistry laboratories to be doing this routinely!

- How big a sample did the investigators use? Did they really use a sample containing as few as 12 subjects? Or perhaps they do not even reveal how many subjects were used! Hedlund and Vieweg (1979) summarized the results of nine reliability studies for a well-known method of measuring severity of depression—the Hamilton Rating Scale for Depression. Two of the studies apparently did not report sample sizes. Of the other seven, the reported sample sizes are 7, 128, 70, 26, 90, 193, 53 and 40. This variability in sample size suggests that it had been given very little serious thought by several of the nine investigating teams. Sample sizes are all too often embarrassingly low.

- An issue related to sample size is the estimation of the standard error or of a confidence interval for the stated reliability or repeatability coefficients. Investigators would probably soon realize the importance of adequate sample sizes if they were to report standard errors routinely.

- Have the authors of the report given sufficient detail for you to replicate their study if you wished? Do they give you enough information for you to attempt to replicate their statistical analysis? How did they calculate their coefficients of reliability and corresponding standard errors? Did they look for outliers? Can you see anything in the data, or their summaries of the data, which might lead you to cast doubt on the validity of their analyses? It would often be very useful to see the authors' raw data, but that is only possible in exceptional cases.

FURTHER READING

Bland, M. and Altman, D.G. (1986). Statistical methods for assessing agreement between two methods of clinical measurement. *Lancet* **i**, 307–10.

Fleiss, J.L. (1981). *Statistical methods for rates and proportions* (Chapter 13). New York: Wiley. (2nd edition.)

Streiner, D.L. and Norman, G.R. (1989). *Health measurement scales. A practical guide to their development and use.* Oxford: Oxford University Press.

EXERCISES

1 Calculate a kappa coefficient for each of the following two-way tables. The observed agreement is 90% in all tables. How do you interpret your findings?

(a)

		Doctor 2	
		Yes	*No*
	Yes	80	5
Doctor 1			
	No	5	10

(b)

		Doctor 2	
		Yes	*No*
	Yes	50	5
Doctor 1			
	No	5	40

(c)

		Doctor 2	
		Yes	*No*
	Yes	80	10
Doctor 1			
	No	0	10

(d)

		Doctor 2	
		Yes	*No*
	Yes	50	10
Doctor 1			
	No	0	40

(e)

		Doctor 2	
		Yes	*No*
	Yes	90	5
Doctor 1			
	No	5	0

(f)

		Doctor 2	
		Yes	*No*
	Yes	90	10
Doctor 1			
	No	0	0

2 In the field of human genetics it is common to assess the heritability of quantitative characteristics by calculating intra-class correlations on samples of monozygotic (identical) and dizygotic (non-identical) twins. If a characteristic is genetically inherited one would expect the similarity (correlation) between identical twins to be higher than that for the non-identical ones. The following 12 pairs of finger ridge counts provides an example of such data from a sample of female identical twins (Newman *et al.*, 1937). Determine the intra-class correlation and its 95% confidence interval.

71, 71	79, 82	105, 99	115, 114	76, 70	83, 82
114, 113	57, 44	114, 113	94, 91	75, 83	76, 72

3　Display 3.15 contains data on measures of lung function: peak expiratory flow rate (PEFR) assessed using a Wright peak flow meter (from Bland and Altman, 1986). Investigate the repeatability and reliability of the PEFR using these data. Calculate the intra-class correlation and corresponding 95% confidence interval. Now introduce an outlier by replacing the first observation for subject 1 (494) by 4944, and repeat your analysis.

Subject	First	Second
1	494	490
2	395	397
3	516	512
4	434	401
5	476	470
6	557	611
7	413	415
8	442	431
9	650	638
10	433	429
11	417	420
12	656	633
13	267	275
14	478	492
15	178	165
16	423	372
17	427	421

DISPLAY 3.15 PEFR (in litres/min) measured with the Wright peak flow meter (from Altman and Bland, 1986)

4　Calculate the reliability for each of the following clinical psychometric tests:

(a) Standard error of measurement = 5; standard deviation = 20
(b) Standard error of measurement = 5; standard deviation = 10
(c) Standard error of measurement = 5; standard deviation = 5
(d) Standard error of measurement = 2; standard deviation = 10
(e) Standard error of measurement = 3; standard deviation = 15

5 Calculate the standard error of measurement (repeatability) for each of the following tests:

(a) Reliability $= 0.90$; standard deviation $= 10$
(b) Reliability $= 0.80$; standard deviation $= 20$
(c) Reliability $= 0.70$; standard deviation $= 20$
(d) Reliability $= 0.50$; standard deviation $= 20$

Sampling and Estimation | 4

4.1 INTRODUCTION

If we know that the average systolic blood pressure of 50 young men is 135 mm Hg what can we say about the mean systolic blood pressure of *all* young men? If a drug is found to alleviate pain in 16 out of a sample of 20 patients suffering from arthritis, what percentage of *all* such patients might be expected to experience the same effect? Using information gathered on samples of patients to draw conclusions about populations is one of the main aims of many statistical analyses. The process, usually known as ***statistical inference***, requires consideration of how the sample was actually selected and how samples of observations vary. Both topics were introduced in Chapter 2 and are now taken up in more detail. Informative summaries of the sample observations are an additional important part of the process, and several methods are described in Section 4.3.

4.2 RANDOM SAMPLING

In Section 2.3 we stressed the importance of ensuring that the ***sampled*** population from which we have obtained our subjects for observation is as close as possible to that of the ***target*** population about which we want to draw conclusions. We also stressed that the sample should be drawn from the sampled population in an objective and unbiased way. It should be representative of the population as a whole. The best way of achieving this is through the use of a ***random*** sampling mechanism. Random sampling implies that whether a subject finishes up in the sample is determined by ***chance***; there is no way of predicting which particular subjects will be in the sample. A familiar example is dealing a hand of playing cards. The dealer should have thoroughly shuffled the pack, without being able to see the identity of any of the cards, prior to dealing. The card player receives, for example, a sample of five of the possible 52 cards and the identity of these five cards is completely determined by chance.

Dealing a hand of playing cards is, in fact, an example of a particular type of random sampling mechanism: **simple random sampling**. The word 'simple' implies that we can enumerate all the possible samples which might be drawn and that the probability of obtaining any one of them is equal to that of any other (i.e. the probabilities are all equal). With a pack of 52 there are 2 598 960 different possible hands of five cards. The probability of obtaining any one of them is therefore 1 in 2 598 960.

Consider a slightly easier example. Suppose we have a small group of six patients with a rare disease, and suppose that we wish to select two of them at random in order to try out a novel form of treatment. We will give these patients one-letter names as follows:

A   B   C   D   E   F

The possibilities for our sample of two patients are quite easy to list and are as follows:

AB   AC   AD   AE   AF
BC   BD   BE   BF   CD
CE   CF   DE   DF   EF

We have a choice of 15 possible samples. If we were to choose one of these 15 samples completely at random then we would be using a simple random sampling scheme and the probability of obtaining any one of these samples would be 1/15.

The use of simple random sampling implies that each *subject* has the same probability of being selected for the sample. The reverse, however, is not necessarily true. Saying that each subject has the same probability of being sampled does *not* necessarily imply that the sampling mechanism follows a simple random sampling procedure. It would be an example of a random sampling procedure, but may be of another type. We will illustrate this with another example. Suppose we have a list of, say, 100 subjects from which samples are to be taken (this list is called a **sampling frame**) and suppose that the subjects in this list each has a unique three-figure numerical code, starting at 001, as follows:

001   002   003   004   005   006   007   008   009   010
011   012   013   014   015   016   017   018   019   020

021	022	023	024	025	026	027	028	029	030
031	032	033	034	035	036	037	038	039	040
041	042	043	044	045	046	047	048	049	050
051	052	053	054	055	056	057	058	059	060
061	062	063	064	065	066	067	068	069	070
071	072	073	074	075	076	077	078	079	080
081	082	083	084	085	086	087	088	089	090
091	092	093	094	095	096	097	098	099	100

Now suppose that we wish to select a sample of 10 subjects for further investigation. A simple way of doing this is to select *at random* one of the first 10 subjects (i.e. one of the first row of numbers) and then to systematically select every tenth subject following the first one to be selected (in this case, all numbers in the column of the first to be selected). Suppose we had initially selected subject 005, then our sample would be

005 015 025 035 045 055 065 075 085 095

If we had initially selected subject 010, it would be

010 020 030 040 050 060 070 080 090 100

These are examples of **systematic random samples**. Each subject has the same probability of being selected, but each of the possible samples does not. Ten of the possible samples each have a probability of 1/10 of being selected, all the others have a probability of 0. An example of the latter is

010 030 023 045 033 056 069 071 075 079

To see why this is so, note that it is impossible, for example, for both subjects 010 and 030 to turn up in the same sample when using this sampling mechanism.

What other forms of random sampling might be used? Perhaps the most common is a **stratified random sample**. Here we divide our sampled population into distinct groups or strata. These could be men and women, different age bands, social classes, and so on. Having chosen our strata we then proceed to take, for example, a simple random sample from each of these strata separately. The proportion of subjects sampled from each strata (the **sampling fraction**) might be constant across all of the samples (ensuring that the overall sample has the same composition as the original population) or we might decide that one or more strata might have a higher representation. Returning to the above table of 100 numerical codes, each row might represent one of ten equally sized strata. Now if we chose one subject (number) at random from each of the rows, this would provide an example of a stratified sample. Another commonly used sampling mechanism is *cluster sampling*. We might, for example, take a sample of clinics and investigate all patients attending each of the sampled clinics. Finally, it is possible to sample in two or more stages. Having selected a random sample of clinics it is often convenient then to select a random sample of patients from within each of the sampled clinics.

One particularly useful form of two-stage sampling that has been used in surveys designed to estimate prevalence (particularly in psychiatry) is called *double sampling*. Here we first select an initial sample at random and carry out some preliminary screening test on all of those sampled. This might be a psychiatric questionnaire (the GHQ mentioned in Chapter 3, for example) or be a simple physical examination such as a chest X-ray. We then classify the sample into two mutually exclusive groups: test positive and test negative. Finally we take a random sample from each of these two groups and proceed with a much more detailed medical investigation of those finally selected. In a survey of the prevalence of psychiatric illness, for example, we might get a sample of people from the community of interest to complete the GHQ. On the basis of their GHQ scores each subject is then classified as GHQ +ve (probably a case) or GHQ −ve (probably not a case). On the assumption that the majority of respondents will be GHQ −ve, we then might choose to optimize our resources by proceeding with a detailed psychiatric interview with all of the GHQ +ve subjects but with a sample of, say, 1 in 4, of the GHQ −ve subjects.

Why have we spent so much time explaining different random sampling methods? The major reason is that many of the statistical procedures described in this and the other chapters are based on the assumption that we have used a simple random sample. It probably does not matter if a systematic random sample has been used instead but if stratified or cluster sampling schemes have been used then it is important that the statistical analysis takes account of this fact. In any particular example, the investigators must be completely explicit about the way in which their samples were chosen, and you should always check the report of a survey or other investigation involving taking samples by asking the following questions:

- Do the authors clearly define the sampled population?

- Do the authors discuss similarities and possible differences between their sampled population and a stated target population?

- Do the authors report what sampling mechanism has been used?

- Is the sampling mechanism random? (If not, then why not?)

- Exactly what sort of random sampling has been used?

- Do the methods of data analysis make allowances for the sampling mechanism used?

What if the investigators have made no attempt at random sampling? Suppose they have simply made use of a consecutive series of 50 patients attending a particular doctor's clinic complaining of chest pains, for example. They may be consecutive patients from two or three clinics. Suppose that a disease is so rare that we do not even have the luxury of sampling—we simply base our study on the 20 patients we can get access to. Many, if not the majority, of the studies reported in medical journals are of this type. The data are usually reported and analysed, however, as if they had arisen from a single simple random sample. The problem here is that we have lost the vital link between a precisely defined random sampling scheme and the appropriate method of statistical inference.

In these circumstances should we therefore abandon statistical inference? Probably not (and even statisticians, including the present authors, proceed with the process), but we should always be very wary of taking our results too seriously. The basis of our inferences has been severely weakened (a purist might say 'destroyed'). Basically we are starting our inferences by saying 'If we pretend that we have a random sample, then ...'. The word 'pretend' has been put in deliberately—it is not an assumption, because we *know* that random sampling has not been used! In the end we have to accept that we are using statistical inference as a guide, as a way of helping make sense out of data, and that our inferences are really based on judgement, not on probabilities.

4.3 THE DESCRIPTION OF SAMPLES

Having obtained a sample of observations from a population by some sampling scheme, an important first step, prior to the inferential process proper, is to describe the observations. This will highlight features that might have implications for the methods to be used, for example, distributions that are skew rather than symmetric, or identify observations that might unduly influence the procedure, so called **statistical outliers**.

Frequency distributions

Let us return once again to Chapter 3's Scottish clinician wrestling with her attempts to discover the implications of maternal drinking for the birth weight of babies. She has studied a sample of 100 women, collected information about the amount of alcohol consumed during pregnancy and weighed their babies. We have already described how the doctor might investigate the correlation or association between the two variables (Section 3.5). We have also described the use of simple summary statistics to indicate typical values and variability of the measures (Sections 3.4 and 3.6). Let us, for the moment, concentrate on further methods of describing the distribution of birth weights.

We start with a **frequency distribution table**, produced by counting the number of observations that fall into each of a number of categories of birth weight. Display 4.2 shows such a table resulting from grouping the birth weights in Display 4.1 into 50g intervals. As we have previously noted, an unsorted table of numbers such as Display 4.1 is not very informative. In Display 4.2, however, it is readily seen that nearly all of the birth weights lie between 2901 and 3100g, with most lying in the interval 3001 to 3050g. Frequency distribution tables are often displayed graphically in the form of a **histogram** as is shown in Display 4.3 (a further example of such a diagram was given earlier in Chapter 2). When a histogram is used to describe the frequency distribution of a data set, it must be remembered that it is the *area* of the rectangle that is being used to represent a frequency. This point is especially pertinent when considering frequency distributions where the class intervals are *not* of equal width. In such situations it is usually necessary to make appropriate adjustments to the histogram in order that the areas of the rectangles remain in proper proportion to one another.

The problem can be illustrated using the age distributing of all deaths in the USA in 1967, shown in Display 4.4. The age intervals used in this display vary in width from one year (0 to 1 year), to 20

Alcohol (g/wk)	Birth weight (g)	Alcohol (g/wk)	Birth weight (g)
0.00	22.12	3054.81	36.99
43.61	2985.33	2963.44	2990.08
23.24	3065.06	28.58	2944.48
47.30	2964.24	44.21	3121.59
54.24	3007.31	39.65	3029.29
40.33	2927.81	29.69	3035.09
61.82	2943.95	28.61	2808.56
26.09	3120.76	39.62	2990.41
29.79	3087.01	37.66	3089.72
9.26	3042.77	9.93	2964.43
31.64	3101.88	20.66	3043.86
27.76	2890.91	32.17	3159.40
46.15	3020.81	40.84	2946.22
18.18	2993.16	0.00	3071.80
32.58	2947.87	0.00	3010.92
16.06	3040.08	46.61	3167.12
40.72	2987.59	19.49	3075.75
29.26	3121.01	19.65	3029.35
25.76	3005.80	16.04	3071.57
38.26	2949.70	29.13	3053.51
26.92	2996.86	43.26	3043.33
21.07	3128.51	39.61	2992.79
34.55	3054.22	12.55	3079.19
14.52	3015.76	6.76	2911.05
43.64	3021.06	36.61	3026.80
29.56	3007.67	38.02	2896.60
20.75	3095.09	37.66	3077.90
32.63	2905.34	33.14	3247.51
30.69	3032.13	12.68	2986.56
27.86	3014.80	48.53	3026.42
0.00	3049.62	8.86	3071.21
11.81	3056.25	16.16	2990.05
0.00	3109.08	56.14	2986.91
12.33	3091.91	48.22	3100.20
43.08	2968.95	0.00	3058.83
30.89	2881.76	0.00	3055.77
0.00	3022.28	0.00	3126.76
35.72	3075.79	18.73	3049.79
47.92	2967.91	32.29	3036.68
15.77	3026.33	21.64	3027.90
14.25	2994.75	20.90	3044.89
29.71	2946.69	27.22	3085.02
24.61	3127.02	39.33	3084.35
21.64	3025.44	0.00	2981.68
34.71	2934.99	4.92	3079.76
25.71	2953.80	0.00	3014.39
7.72	2956.15	26.95	2938.60
11.51	3071.87	23.17	3006.84
7.03	3101.65	11.59	3054.89
55.74	2930.65	38.22	3011.05

DISPLAY 4.1 Material alcohol consumption and birth weight measurements

Interval	Frequency
2801–2850	1
2851–2900	3
2901–2950	12
2951–3000	19
3001–3050	29
3051–3100	23
3101–3150	10
3151–3200	2
3201–3250	1

DISPLAY 4.2 Frequency distribution table for the birth weights in Display 4.1

years (25–44 years). Before constructing the corresponding histogram for these data, all group intervals need to be scaled so that they are comparable. Since one year is the smallest interval in the distribution it is convenient to scale all other intervals to this level. So, to retain the proper proportion in area for the histogram, an interval that is, say, 20 times as wide as the smallest interval must, when graphed, have a height 1/20th of the frequency of that interval. In other words, number of deaths *per year* is used to construct the appropriate histogram, see Display 4.5.

An alternative method of graphically displaying a frequency distribution table is the *frequency polygon*. In this case a plot of category mid-point against category frequency is made and the points joined by a series of straight lines. Display 4.6 shows the frequency polygon for all the birth weight data, but this type of figure is most useful when the frequency distributions of two or more data sets are to be compared. Suppose, for example, that the clinician who had collected the birth weight data had also recorded the age of the mother, and wished to compare the birth weights of babies born to 'younger' mothers (those between 16 and 28 years) with the birth weight of babies of 'older' mothers (those over 28 years old). The frequency distributions found in each case are shown

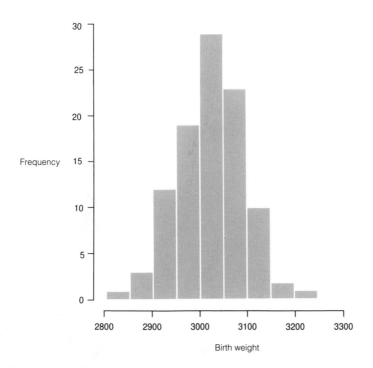

DISPLAY 4.3 Histogram of birthweights in Display 4.1

Age at death (y)	Class limits (y)	Midpoint of interval (y)	Width of interval (y)	Number of deaths	Deaths per year of age
Under 1	0–1	0.5	1	79 028	79 028
1–4	1–5	3	4	13 506	3 377
5–9	5–10	7.5	5	8 809	1 762
10–14	10–15	12.5	5	8 084	1 617
15–24	15–25	20	10	37 706	3 771
25–44	25–45	35	20	108 825	5 441
45–64	45–65	55	20	459 203	22 960
65–74	65–75	70	10	437 919	43 792
75–84	75–85	80	10	469 669	46 967
85+	85–100	92.5	15	227 987	15 199

DISPLAY 4.4 Deaths in the USA recorded in the year 1967

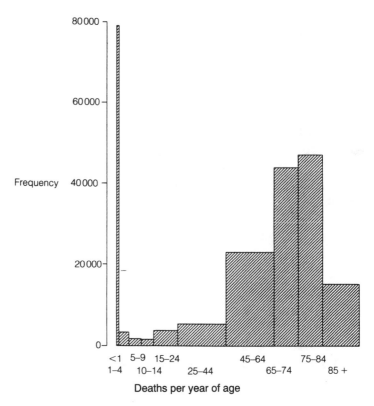

DISPLAY 4.5 Histogram for the deaths recorded in Display 4.4

in Display 4.7. The corresponding frequency polygons can be conveniently displayed on the same diagram as shown in Display 4.8. This diagram suggests that babies born to older mothers tend to have higher birth weights.

Although histograms and frequency polygons often give a very useful graphical representation of a set of data, they do involve some loss of information compared to having the original observations, since the individual observations are no longer available after the groups in the frequency distribution table have been formed. A procedure which overcomes this possible disadvantage is the *stem-and-leaf plot*. With this type of diagram, a graphical display of the frequency distribution of the observation is combined with the retention of the separate observations. This approach is illustrated

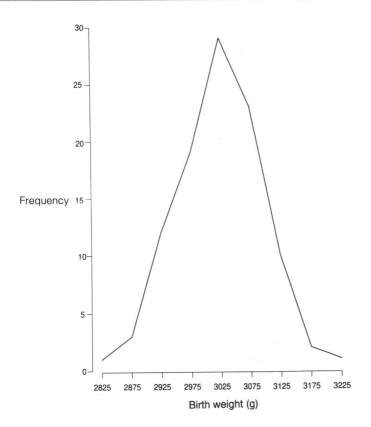

DISPLAY 4.6 Frequency polygon for birth weight data in Display 4.1

in Display 4.9 using the ages of the mothers in the birth weight study. The stem-and-leaf is very simple to produce and is really nothing more than a tally of the observations written out in a particularly helpful format. Not all useful statistical procedures involve a lot of difficult arithmetic!

Before moving on to consider more concise ways of describing and summarizing a set of data it may be helpful to make some more general comments about graphical presentations of data, in particular to issue some caveats! In the main, graphics are very helpful, particularly in presenting numerical material to the non-numerically minded. Unfortunately graphical displays are occasionally designed to mislead the unwary, often with some success. Two examples will

(a) Younger mothers (16–28 years)

Interval	Frequency
2801–2850	1
2851–2900	2
2901–2950	8
2951–3000	12
3001–3050	16
3051–3100	11
3101–3150	3
3151–3200	0
3201–3250	0
Total	53

(b) Older mothers (>28 years)

Interval	Frequency
2801–2850	0
2851–2900	1
2901–2950	4
2951–3000	7
3001–3050	13
3051–3100	12
3101–3150	7
3151–3200	2
3201–3250	1
Total	47

DISPLAY 4.7 Frequency distributions for birth weight by age of mother

suffice to illustrate the possibilities. Consider, for example, the 'shrinking doctors' shown in Display 4.10 (reproduced from Tufte, 1983). This diagram is being used to highlight the decline in the percentage of doctors devoted solely to family practice. Such a decline is occurring, but this diagram exaggerates the effect by using the decrease in the *area* of the doctor icon to represent the decrease in a single variable. Further exaggeration is achieved by the overlaid perspective and the incorrect horizontal spacing of the data.

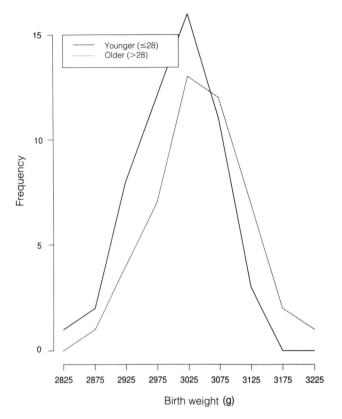

DISPLAY 4.8 Frequency polygons of birth weights of children of younger and older mothers

As a further example of a graph which is not completely honest, consider Display 4.11. This graph shows the death ratio per million from cancer of the breast for several periods over the last three decades. As presented here, the rates appear to show a rather alarming increase. But when redrawn so that the vertical scale starts at zero, as shown in Display 4.12, the increase in the breast cancer death rate is seen to be rather less depressing. This example illustrates that when drawing graphs undue exaggeration or comparison of the scales must be avoided.

Five-number summaries and box-and-whisker plots

One of the most useful methods of summarizing sample information is to represent it by a *five-number summary*; the five numbers being

$N = 100$ Median $= 3026.61$

Low $= 2808.56$

Quartiles $= 2985.95, 3071.84$

288	2
289	17
290	5
291	1
292	8
293	159
294	44678
295	046
296	34489
297	
298	25778
299	0003357
300	6778
301	11456
302	1125667899
303	257
304	03345
305	004455669
306	5
307	12226689
308	0457
309	025
310	0229
311	
312	112779
313	
314	
315	9
316	7

High $= 3247.51$

Key: The stem represents the number of tens; the leaves are units

The minimum and maximum values are not included in the stem-and-leaf plot, to avoid an excess of blank lines.

DISPLAY 4.9 Stem-and-leaf plots for birth weight data

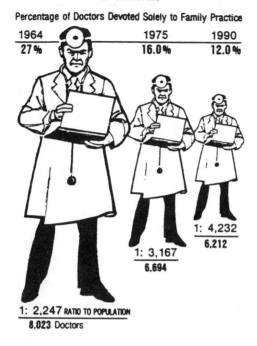

THE SHRINKING FAMILY DOCTOR
In California

Percentage of Doctors Devoted Solely to Family Practice

1964	1975	1990
27%	16.0%	12.0%

1: 4,232
6.212

1: 3,167
6.694

1: 2,247 RATIO TO POPULATION
8,023 Doctors

DISPLAY 4.10 Tufte's shrinking doctor example (taken with permission from Tufte, 1983)

the lowest value, the lower quartile, the median, the upper quartile and, finally the highest value. Associated with this five-number summary is the ***box-and-whisker plot*** (often shortened to box plot). A box plot for all of the birth weight data is given in Display 4.13. Here the median is used to indicate location (central value), the range of the upper and lower quartiles to indicate typical spread (dispersion), and the maximum and minimum values of the data (after exclusion of the one or more outliers defined in the manner described below) are also given to complete the picture. To construct this display a box is drawn with ends at the upper and lower quartiles of the data and a crossbar at the median value. Next a line is drawn from each end of the box to the most remote observation (i.e. the lowest and highest values), again excluding the outlying observations, forming the two whiskers. Finally, the positions of the outliers are indicated using a separate symbol (*, for example).

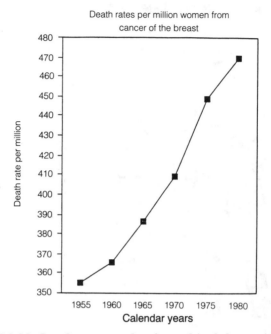

DISPLAY 4.11 Another example of graphical deception

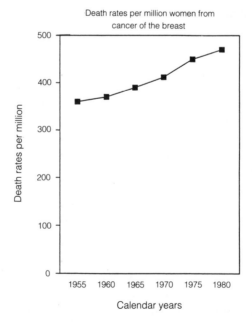

DISPLAY 4.12 Redrawn version of Display 4.11

The procedure for the detection of the outliers involves the definition of two limits, with observations outside those limits being considered outliers. The limits are defined and the procedure illustrated in Display 4.15 using anxiety scores from a sample of patients attending a dental clinic for a wisdom tooth extraction (Display 4.14). Display 4.16 provides a further illustration of the box plot using the anxiety data.

If we see that the distance between the median and the upper quartile is greater than the corresponding distance between the median and lower quartile and, similarly the distance from the median to the highest value is *greater* than the distance from the median to the lowest value, then this is evidence of asymmetry in the distribution. This would also, of course, have been detected on looking at a histogram or stem-and-leaf plot. This is an example of ***positive skewness***. On the other hand, if the two distances above the median had been lower than those below, then this would be evidence of ***negative skewness***. Checking for skewness is one of the more important aspects of a preliminary data analysis. This is because our methods of statistical inference (e.g. confidence interval construction) often assume that the data are Normally distributed, see next section.

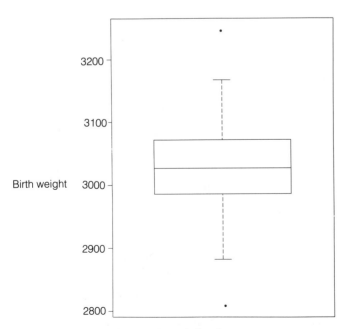

DISPLAY 4.13 Box plot for birth weight data

Women:

28.8	29.4	28.1	27.9	31.8
30.0	31.3	28.2	28.7	30.7
30.3	29.4	31.1	29.3	27.3
31.8	31.9	28.5	30.6	25.4
29.9	30.6	27.7	34.4	39.0

Men:

38.7	35.5	32.4	31.1	32.8
27.4	27.7	34.0	28.2	35.3
33.6	29.8	30.7	30.1	34.4
29.4	32.0	30.2	33.7	32.5
35.8	29.8	34.7	27.4	20.0

DISPLAY 4.14 Anxiety in dental patients

The five-number summary of the anxiety data is:

Minimum:	20.00
Lower quartile (LQ):	28.70
Median:	30.45
Upper quartile (UQ):	32.50
Maximum:	39.00

Inter-quartile range (IQR): $32.50 - 28.70$
                                        $= 3.80$

Cut-offs used to define outliers are

$$LQ - 1.5 \times IQR \quad \text{and} \quad UQ + 1.5 \times IQR$$

Here these limits are

$$28.70 - 1.5 \times 3.80 = 23.00 \quad \text{and} \quad 32.50 + 1.50 \times 3.80 = 38.20$$

There are three values which are outside of these limits, with values of 20.0, 38.7 and 39.0. These are the outliers.

DISPLAY 4.15 Definition of outliers, using anxiety scores as an example

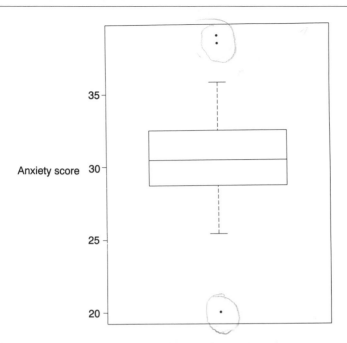

DISPLAY 4.16 Box plot with outliers for anxiety data

Box-plots are often particularly useful for the *comparison* of data sets. Display 4.17, for example, shows the separate box-plots of the anxiety scores of male and female dental patients. (Note that there are now only two outliers, one in each group. The value of 38.7 is not defined to be an outlier when women are considered as a separate group.) At a glance, we can see if there is evidence of group differences in the medians (typical values), whether there is constant dispersion or the variability (and, in particular, whether the variability as measured by the IQR) is increasing as the median increases. We can also see whether the samples are approximately symmetrical and, if not, whether they are positively or negatively skewed. Finally, we might also see evidence of outliers. Quite a lot from a single graph!

4.4 REFERENCE RANGES AND THE NORMAL DISTRIBUTION

If the frequency distribution of the individual's measurements is more-or-less symmetrical it can often be approximated by the

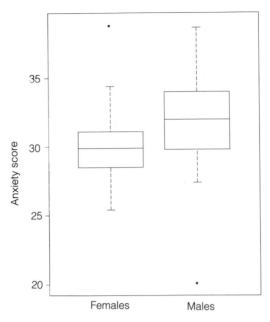

DISPLAY 4.17 Separate box plots for anxiety scores of male and female dental patients

Normal distribution introduced briefly in Chapter 2. (Some relevant properties of the Normal distribution are illustrated in Display 4.18). If this is the case then we can simply calculate the sample mean and sample standard deviation and claim that 95% of the individuals will lie within approximately two standard deviations either side of the mean. That is, 5% will lie outside of this region. In the context of diagnostic tests applied to samples of apparently healthy individuals, this provides a rough and ready guide to the test's *reference range*, with an 'abnormal' test result being defined as one that does not lie within the central 95% region.

Reference ranges are most commonly associated with tests from clinical chemistry but it is possible, of course, to construct such intervals for many other characteristics of interest, for example, blood pressure measurements and even GHQ scores. Any patient who is suspected of suffering from a given illness then has his or her test result compared with those provided by the reference sample. If the score falls outside the expected range for the central 95% of 'normal' scores then it is labelled as 'abnormal' and interpreted as an indication of pathology. In the case of a GHQ score, it might be thought silly to look at the bottom end of the range (people who are

Normal distributions are a family of symmetrical 'bell-shaped' curves. They are all of the same basic shape, but are distinguished by (and are completely described by) their mean value (position) and standard deviation (spread). Display 4.19(c) provides two examples. The *standard Normal distribution* is a special case that has a mean equal to 0 and a standard deviation of 1.

If a random variable is Normally distributed then the probability that a randomly selected value will fall within one standard deviation of the mean (that is, will have a value between $\mu - \sigma$ and $\mu + \sigma$, where μ is the distribution's mean, and σ its standard deviation) is 0.683. The probability that it will lie within two standard deviations of the mean is 0.954 and, finally, the probability that it will be within three standard deviations of the mean is 0.997. *A value outside this range is very rare.* In the case of the standard Normal distribution, the probability of getting a value between -2 and $+2$, for example, is therefore 0.954 (here $\mu = 0$ and $\sigma = 1$ so $\mu - 2\sigma = -2$ and $\mu + 2\sigma = +2$).

The middle 95% of Normally-distributed values fall within the range $\mu - 1.96\sigma$ to $\mu + 1.96\sigma$ (in the case of the standard Normal distribution, within the range -1.96 to $+1.96$). The middle 99% of the values fall within the range $\mu - 2.58\sigma$ to $\mu + 2.58\sigma$ (again, in the case of the standard Normal distribution, -2.58 to $+2.58$). Remember that, if 95% of the values fall within a given range then it automatically follows that 5% fall outside of it. Because of the symmetrical nature of the distribution it also means that equal numbers (2.5%) fall below the interval and above it.

DISPLAY 4.18 Characteristics of the Normal distribution

apparently too well-adjusted!) and it might, therefore, be more sensible to ask whether the GHQ score obtained lies in the *top* 5% of the reference range. The same would also apply to biochemical markers of heart muscle damage such as creatine kinase. Blood pressure, on the other hand, might be pathologically low (hypotension) as well as pathologically high (hypertension). The interpretation of reference ranges is fraught with difficulties—not least the decision concerning who to include in a sample of supposedly normal healthy individuals—but, it is still very useful to have an understanding of variability between individuals. Although invoking the Normal distribution in this way is frequently a justified and convenient descriptive device, it is not *always* possible; GHQ scores, for example, are usually highly skewed.

The importance of the Normal distribution does not end solely with its use for the description of the pattern of relative frequency of individual measurements; the distribution is also very important in describing how samples vary and in the derivation of *sampling distributions*, a topic that was discussed briefly in Chapter 2 and is now considered in more detail in the following section.

4.5 SAMPLING DISTRIBUTIONS

The existence of sampling variation implies that it is not possible to make *definite* claims about a population on the basis of information gathered from a sample, (i.e. we cannot assume the equality of a sample statistic and a population parameter). Knowing that the average systolic blood pressure in a sample of 50 young men in 135 mm Hg does not allow us to say that the mean systolic blood pressure of *all* young men is 135 mm Hg. A drug that is found to alleviate pain in 16 out of a sample of 20 patients suffering from arthritis, will not necessarily have a similar effect in 80% of all such patients. The results from a single sample are subject to *statistical uncertainty*, and statements made about a population on the basis of sample values need to reflect this uncertainty by being couched in terms of probabilities. In this way the uncertainty is quantified.

Let us begin by assuming that we are eager to learn something about the average systolic blood pressure in our ubiquitous population of young men. A representative sample of 50 individuals from the population is found to have a mean of 135.0 mm Hg and a standard deviation of 10.6 mm Hg. We know that, because of sampling variation, the mean of the population is very unlikely to be exactly equal to the sample mean, but it might be hoped that it is, perhaps, not too far away. The sample mean is said to be an *estimator* of the population's value, although it is not the only way that the population mean could be estimated from sample values. Why not, for example, estimate the population mean by the sample median? The answer is that the sample mean can be shown to have a number of desirable properties that make it a 'good' estimator of the population mean. In particular, the value of the sample mean is, on average, very likely to be closer to the population value than is any other estimate. This does not mean that the sample mean will *always* be closer, only that there is a higher probability that this will be so. (Note, however, that in the presence of outliers, it can be shown that the sample median is the better of the two estimates since as mentioned in the previous chapter it is largely unaffected by such observations). Here we will assume that we have no outliers so that the sample mean is the estimator of choice.

Returning to the systolic blood pressure example, 135.0 mm Hg is the estimate of the population mean obtained from our 50 observations. But on its own this figure is not really of great value; the sample mean is an imprecise estimate of the population value and needs to be accompanied by some measure of the imprecision. What is really needed is a *range* (interval) of possible values for the population mean, together with some measure of how confident we are that the interval does, in fact, contain the population value. If the sample size is reasonably large, then such a range of values, a *confidence interval*, can be found from consideration of the sample mean using methods analogous to those described in Section 2.4. The basis of the procedure is what is known as the *sampling distribution* of the sample mean. To illustrate what is meant by this term, consider a population of values of systolic blood pressures. Assume that these values have a Normal distribution with mean 140 mm Hg and standard deviation 20 mm Hg. Suppose repeated random samples of some particular size, say 50, are selected and for each the sample mean calculated. What does the distribution of these mean values look like? Not surprisingly perhaps the distribution is Normal, but what is its mean and standard deviation? The answer is that the mean of the sampling distribution of sample means is the same as that of the original distribution (here 140 mm Hg), but the standard deviation of the sampling distribution is the original standard deviation divided by the square root of the sample size. The process is illustrated in Display 4.19(a), which shows histograms of four samples of size 50 from the relevant Normal distribution, and Display 4.19(b), which gives the histogram of the sample means of 100 samples of size 50. Display 4.19(c) shows the theoretical sampling distribution of the sample mean of samples of size 50, together with the original Normal distribution.

The standard deviation of the sampling distribution of sample means is generally known as the *standard error of the mean*. It can be estimated by dividing the sample standard deviation by the square root of the sample size, and from the estimated standard error we can then determine the required 95% confidence interval for the population mean from the observed mean, ± 1.96 standard errors. Details of the calculation for the systolic blood pressure of

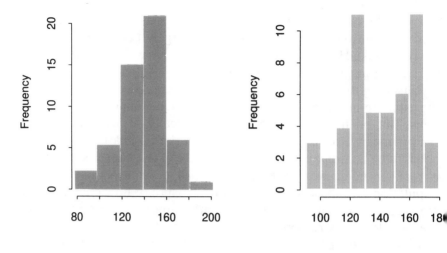

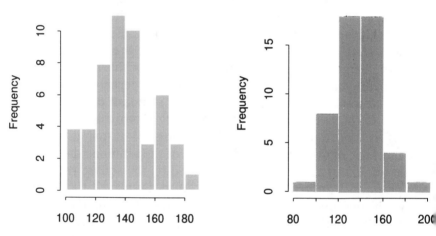

(a) Four samples of size 50 from a Normal distribution

DISPLAY 4.19(a–c) Sampling distribution of the sample mean when sampling from a Normal distribution

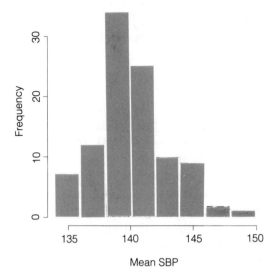

(b) Histogram of means of 100 samples size 50 from a Normal distribution

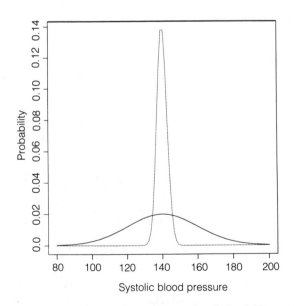

(c) Sample distribution of sample mean and original Normal distribution

young men example are given in Display 4.20. (In the case of small sample sizes, the confidence interval given in this display will need to be modified—see the discussion of the t distribution in the Postscript following Chapter 6.)

Note that for reasonably large samples, at least, the Normality of the sampling distribution of the sample mean remains approximately true even when the individual values themselves are *not* Normally distributed. Displays 4.21(a) and 4.21(b) illustrate this point. The first of these displays shows four samples of size 50 from what is known as a uniform distribution in the interval (0, 1) (that is, all possible values between 0 and 1 have the same probability). The second display shows the histogram obtained from 100 samples of size 50 from this uniformly distributed population. The importance of the Normal distribution in statistical inference rests on the fact that many sample statistics can be shown to be Normally distributed even when the individual observations are far from Normal. The example which we have already encountered in Chapter 2, for instance, involves the Normality of a sample proportion when the observations themselves can only take the two values of, say, 0 (healthy) and 1 (ill).

Suppose that we have obtained a sample of 50 individuals and estimated their mean and standard deviation. The sample mean is 135.0 and the sample standard deviation is 10.6.

We first calculate (estimate) the standard error of the mean, which is the above standard deviation divided by the square root of the sample size (that is, 10.6/7.07). The standard error of the mean is therefore 1.50, approximately.

A 95% confidence interval for the mean is constructed as follows. The lower limit is given by the sample mean minus 1.96 standard errors (that is $135.0 - 1.96 \times 1.50$). The upper limit is the sample mean plus 1.96 standard errors ($135.0 + 1.96 \times 1.50$). The resulting values are usually separated by a comma and placed within parentheses. The required confidence interval is therefore (132.06, 137.94).

The corresponding 99% confidence interval is $135.0 - 2.58 \times 1.50$ to $135.0 + 2.58 \times 1.50$, or (131.13, 138.87).

DISPLAY 4.20 Calculation of the standard error of a mean and corresponding 95% confidence interval

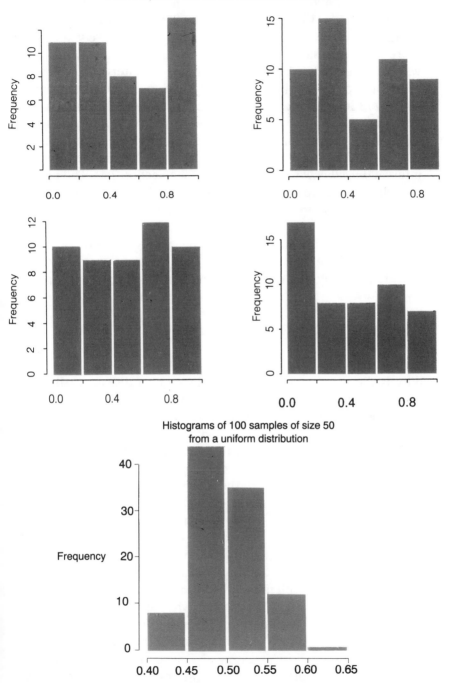

DISPLAY 4.21 Sampling distribution of the sample mean when sampling from a non-Normal distribution

The 95% confidence interval for the mean systolic blood pressure of young men is (132.1, 137.9). There is 95% chance that this interval contains the true value of the population mean. If we wanted to be more confident, say 99%, then the corresponding confidence interval would be (131.1, 138.9). The width of the interval has increased. This is the price that has to be paid for being more certain that the calculated interval includes the value of the population mean. One very important point about confidence intervals must be stressed again: since the population mean is fixed, it is *not* correct to say that the probability is 0.95 or 0.99 that the mean is in the confidence interval *once this has been calculated* (see Section 2.4). The probability value applies to the calculated interval. Such intervals would be expected to contain the true value of the population mean 95 times out of a 100.

The material introduced up to this point will now be used in considering a very important problem in many areas of medical research, namely that of estimating the prevalence of a disease.

4.6 THE ESTIMATION OF THE PREVALENCE OF DISEASES

Why is the estimation of the prevalence of a disease or illness so important? In Chapter 2 we discussed the use of Bayes' theorem in making diagnoses or in the interpretation of the use of screening test results. If your patient has just had a smear test for cancer of the cervix, and you wish to ask her to return for further tests because of a positive result, then it becomes of more than academic importance to you to understand how the probability of having cancer is dependent on the prevalence of the disease, as well as on the characteristics of the smear test. The same applies to a positive test result for HIV antibodies. The patient will probably need advice and counselling. You wish to avoid panic in your patient, and you need to explain that in the case of a rare disease, in particular, most of the positive test results will, in fact, be false positives.

There are, of course, other reasons why we might be interested in the prevalence or incidence of disease. It is obviously vitally important for health-care planners to know the relative frequencies of different diseases in assessing the needs for different types of clinical facility. Studies of the changing rates of incidence of HIV infection (or of AIDS, itself) will, at the very least, give us a rough estimate of the likely need for specialized facilities in the coming years. If we are lucky it might also give us clues about the mode of transmission of the illness, and ways in which we might reduce its rate of spread in the population. Comparison of the prevalence of a particular illness in different countries, or comparing regions within a country, might give us clues to the possible causes. The raised incidence of childhood leukaemia in the vicinity of nuclear power stations is one well-known example. The suspected effects of natural radiation (radon from the underlying rock formations) on other forms of cancer is another. The interpretation of data arising from studies attempting to link suspected environmental hazards with increased risk of disease is a very difficult business, however, and the subject abounds with pitfalls and controversies. Some of these problems will be discussed in the following chapter. Here, however, we shall continue to concentrate on the relatively simple problem of estimating a population proportion.

Our main interest is in prevalence, where this proportion will be based on the number of people who are found to be ill at a particular time or during a particular study period. But two other areas where estimation of a proportion is important should be mentioned. The first involves the *incidence rate* for an illness which is based on the number of people in a sample who develop a particular illness during a fixed time interval, and the second, the *mortality rate* is based on the number of people who die over the period. The statistical principles of estimation of a proportion are the same for all three situations.

One of the problems of prevalence estimation is the assumption that the disease state of a person is black or white: they are either well or they are ill. In reality, there are often many shades of grey. Should we automatically assume that someone with a high blood pressure is ill and in need of care? Is a subject who scores high on the General Health Questionnaire always in need of psychiatric help? Obviously not. There are many transient sources of stress which will influence the symptoms recorded by the GHQ, for example, such as a tomorrow's degree exam, worries about a house purchase, or even a hangover as the result of the previous evening's party. Blood pressure might be raised through anxiety resulting from the simple act of visiting a doctor! It also might be chronically abnormal—either very low or very high—without any apparent ill effects. Even if high test scores for a quantitative indicator of illness always implied pathology, there is still often a problem arising from the imprecise division between health and illness. There is often a unimodal distribution of test scores within a population with no clearly recognizable point on the scale at which one could now say with confidence 'This patient is ill' (implying that a score below this is a sign of good health). The cut-off point distinguishing illness and health is often entirely arbitrary—although it will usually be chosen to optimize the sensitivity and specificity of the test.

Let us begin with a very simple example involving the estimation of the proportion of children under the age of 15 who suffer from asthma, based on finding nine asthma sufferers amongst a simple random sample of 100 children. The required estimate is 0.09. The procedure for finding the standard error of a proportion and constructing an approximate confidence interval was described in Chapter 2 and is shown again in Display 4.22(a). In our asthma example the estimated standard error is 0.03 and the 95% confidence interval (0.03, 0.15). The prevalence of asthma in this population of children could be as high as 15% or as low as 3%.

Now let us look at another example. Suppose we have the results of a thorough psychiatric interview on 100 patients attending a general practice clinic. We have found that 30 of them, say, are diagnosed as suffering from depression. The estimated prevalence of depression is 0.30. Assuming, again, that we have a simple random sample, the standard error of this estimate is again found using the appropriate formula given in Display 4.22(a). The value is 0.046, and the corresponding 95% confidence interval for the prevalence of depression is approximately (0.21, 0.39). Suppose that this sample, instead of arising from simple random sampling, was actually a stratified sample: 70 women and 30 men (reflecting the proportions of men and women visiting the clinic). The stratum proportions are 70/100 (0.70) and 30/100 (0.30), respectively. Of the 70 women, 25 were depressed (prevalence estimate 0.36) and of the 30 men, five were depressed (prevalence estimate 0.17). Using the addition and multiplication rules for combining probabilities given in Section 2.2, the estimate for the sample as a whole is 0.30, as before. But what is its standard error? This is found using the formula in Display 4.22(b). It is 0.045. The 95% confidence interval for the combined prevalence estimate is still (0.21, 0.39).

Finally, consider double sampling. Suppose that the sample of 100 patients had initially been given a simple (and fallible) screening questionnaire to detect depression. 40 patients were classified as screen negative and the other 60 screen negative. The investigator

In all cases the 95% CI is estimated from

$$P - 1.96 \times se(P) \quad \text{to} \quad P + 1.96 \times se(P)$$

where the standard error of the estimate of the proportion, P, depends on the sampling design as follows.

(a) Based on a simple random sample
Sample size $= N$
Estimated prevalence $= P$

$$se(P): \quad sqrt[P(1 - P)/N]$$

(b) Based on Stratified Sampling (with sample counts proportional to strata sizes)
Here we assume that we have only two strata.

Stratum 1:
    Stratum proportion (weight): W_1
    Sample size: N_1
    Number of with disease: D_1
    Estimated prevalence: $P_1 = D_1/N_1$
Stratum 2:
    Stratum proportion (weight): W_2
    Sample size: N_2
    Number of with disease: D_2
    Estimated prevalence: $P_2 = D_2/N_2$

Combined prevalence estimate: $P = W_1 \times P_1 + W_2 \times P_2$

$$se(P): \quad sqrt\{[W_1^2 + P_1(1 - P_1)/N_1] + [W_2^2 + P_2(1 - P_2)/N_2]\}$$

(c) Based on double sampling
Total sample size: N
Number screen+: N_1
Proportion screen+: W_1
Number screen−: N_2
Proportion screen−: W_2
Number screen+ followed-up: M_1
Number diseased: D_1
Proportion diseased: $P_1 = D_1/M_1$
Number screen− followed up: M_2
Number diseased: D_2
Proportion diseased: $P_2 = D_2/M_2$
Overall prevalence (P): $W_1 \times P_1 + W_2 \times P_2$

$$se(P): \quad sqrt\{[W_1^2 \times P_1(1 - P_1)/N_1] + [W_2^2 \times P_2(1 - P_2)/N_2] + (P_1 - P_2)^2 \times W_1 \times W_2/N\}$$

If P_1 is not too dissimilar to P_2 this expression can be simplified to

$$sqrt\{[W_1^2 \times P_1(1 - P_1)/N_1] + [W_2^2 \times P_2(1 - P_2)/N_2]\}$$

as in the stratified sampling example.

DISPLAY 4.22 Standard errors and 95% confidence intervals for estimated proportions

now chose to interview all of the 30 screen +ve patients, but only 20 (33%) of the screen negative ones. Of the 40 screen +ves, 24 were found to be depressed on interview. Of the screen negative patients, two were found to be depressed on interview. Again, using a combination of the addition and multiplication rules of probability described in Section 2.2, the estimated prevalence is 0.30, as before. The standard error is calculated using the formula in Display 4.22(c) and found to be 0.056. The corresponding confidence interval is (0.19, 0.41). The presumed gain in time and cost of not having to interview all the screen −ve patients has only led to a marginal loss in precision of the prevalence estimate.

What if the investigator had collected a haphazard sample of patients by visiting 10–15 family doctors' clinics and interviewing who he happened to meet in the waiting room. What would the standard error be now? We have not got a clue!

FURTHER READING

Abrahamson, J.H. (1988). *Making sense of data: a self-instructional manual on the interpretation of epidemiological data.* Section B (Rates and other measures). Oxford: Oxford University Press.

Gardner, M.J. and Altman, D.G. (1989). *Statistics with confidence.* London: British Medical Journal (Chapters 1 to 4).

EXERCISES

1   The following table gives the mean and standard deviation of heart rates and blood pressures obtained from 566 healthy males in the age range 18–40 years. What do you think the range of the observations will be in each case?

Variable	Mean	SD
Heart rate (bpm)	77.3	12.83
Systolic BP (mm Hg)	128.8	13.05
Diastolic BP (mm Hg)	79.7	9.39
Pulse pressure (mm Hg)	49.1	11.14

2 The data below gives the ages of 25 mothers in a labour ward who had recently been delivered of their first child. Also recorded are the sex of the child and its birth weight in grams. From previous records IQ scores of the mothers are also available.

IQ	BW (grams)	Age (years)	Sex (1 = F, 2 = M)
125	3036	28	1
86	3005	31	1
119	3152	32	1
113	3073	20	2
101	2882	30	1
143	2943	30	1
132	3117	27	2
106	3056	36	2
121	2980	34	2
109	2915	29	1
88	2934	27	2
116	2991	24	1
102	2845	26	1
75	2850	23	1
90	3036	24	2
109	3077	22	2
104	2964	35	2
110	3071	24	1
96	3050	24	2
101	2937	23	1
95	2972	36	1
117	3080	21	2
115	2936	39	2
102	2700	41	1
90	3351	17	2

• Construct a histogram for the birth weights.
• Construct stem-and-leaf plots for age and the IQ scores.
• Construct separate box plots for age and IQ for girls and boys.
• Draw a scatter plot of age (x axis) against birth weight (y axis). Distinguish between boys and girls on your plot.
• Make an informed 'guess' of the value of the correlation coefficient for age and birth weight and check your guess against the calculated value.
• Indicate on the scatter plot any observations that you think may be unduly influencing the value of the correlation between age and birth weight. How do you think the value of the correlation coefficient would change if these observations were removed?

The Search for Associations | 5

5.1 INTRODUCTION

Some of the most difficult, but also most important, questions dealt with by medical researchers concern whether an association exists between a so-called *risk factor* and the incidence of a disease. Does living near a nuclear power station, for example, increase the chance of children developing leukaemia? Does working at a computer terminal for several hours a day increase the risk of a pregnant women having a miscarriage? Does smoking cigarettes cause lung cancer?

The investigation of such topics is part of what is known formally as *epidemiology*, a subject that is also concerned with describing the distribution and size of disease populations (essentially estimating prevalence, see Chapter 4), and providing data essential for the management, evaluation and planning of services. In this chapter, however, our main interest will be in the assessment and inter-pretation of associations between possible risk factors and particular diseases. Two main types of investigation will be described, the *retrospective study* and the *prospective study*. It should be noted here, however, that in general it is extremely difficult to demonstrate unequivocally *causality* with such studies. However strong the evidence for an association, there will almost always be an alter-native explanation for the observed link between the risk factor and the disease, other than simply that the risk factor *causes* the disease. Nevertheless epidemiological studies designed to identify possible etiological factors in the pathogenesis of disease remain extremely important.

5.2 TWO APPROACHES TO UNCOVERING AN ASSOCIATION

Suppose a clinician suspects that consuming large amounts of chocolate leads to an increased risk of depression. There are a number of ways that she might proceed to investigate her suspicion. Here we shall concentrate on the two which are of most importance.

Prospective studies

A prospective study begins with two groups of people, the first contains people exposed to the risk factor of interest, and the second contains people without such exposure. At the outset of the investigation members of both groups are assumed to be disease free. The people in each group are then followed up for some pre-specified period of time, at the end of which estimates of the incidence of the disease in each group are compared in some way (see later). The results of such an investigation can then be summarized in the form of a *2 × 2 contingency table* as shown in Display 5.1.

In terms of our specific example involving eating excess chocolate and depression, the investigation would begin with a group of non-depressed 'chocoholics' and a group of non-depressed people with a more moderate consumption of chocolate. A hypothetical set of data obtained after a number of years follow-up is shown in Display 5.2. From these data we find that the proportion of excessive chocolate eaters with depression it is 65/565 (or 11.5%), whilst that in the moderate chocolate eaters group it is 25/675 (or 3.7%). These two proportions are estimates of the incidence (often also termed *risk*) of depression amongst chocoholics and non-chocoholics respectively. A commonly used procedure to summarize the results of a prospective study is to compare these separate risk estimates by calculating what is known as the *relative risk*. This is simply the ratio of the estimated risks in each group, giving here the value 11.5/3.7 = 3.11. The relative risk tells a clinician how much the risk for a patient with the risk factor is increased, compared to a person without the factor; and quantifies the benefit that might accrue to the patient if the risk factor was removed. So in this example the risk of suffering from depression amongst those people who consume large amounts of chocolate is estimated to be approximately three

(1) Initial stage of a prospective study (counts)

	Disease will develop	Disease will not develop	Total*
Risk factor present	unknown	unknown	$a+b$
Risk factor absent	unknown	unknown	$c+d$
Total	unknown	unknown	$a+b+c+d$

* In terms of the counts subsequently available at the final stage of the study; only the totals $a+b$ and $c+d$ are known since they are fixed by the sampling design.

(2) Final stage of a prospective study (counts)

	Disease present	Disease absent	Total
Risk factor present	a	b	$a+b$
Risk factor absent	c	d	$c+d$
Total	$a+c$	$b+d$	$a+b+c+d$

(3) Diagrammatic representation of a prospective study

DISPLAY 5.1 Prospective studies

times that amongst more moderate chocolate eaters. (Note that the relative risk does *not* directly relate to the probability that someone with the risk factor will develop the disease. The relative risk may be high, but there may still be only a remote chance of a person who has the risk factor contracting the disease, if the disease is rare.)

As we have seen in other chapters any estimate needs to be given a range of values, a confidence interval, to make it useful, and this applies equally to the estimate of relative risk. This is possible, although a little complicated! Details are given in Display 5.3. For the chocolate/depression example the resulting approximate 95% confidence interval is found to be (1.99, 4.90). If both chocoholics

(1) Initial stage of study (counts)

	Depression will develop	Depression will not develop	Total
Chocoholic	unknown	unknown	565
Non-chocoholic	unknown	unknown	675
Total	unknown	unknown	1240

(2) Final stage of a prospective study (counts)

	Depressed	Not depressed	Total
Chocoholic	65	500	565
Non-chocoholic	25	650	675
Total	90	1150	1240

DISPLAY 5.2 Results of a hypothetical prospective study

and moderate chocolate eaters had the same risk of depression the relative risk in the population would be one. The calculated confidence interval gives some evidence that the relative risk is greater than one and therefore that there *is* an increased risk of depression amongst those people who consume excessive amounts of chocolate (but see the section on confounding variables, p. 110).

Retrospective or case-control studies

A retrospective study begins, like the prospective one, with two groups of people. Now, however, one of the groups consists of individuals who have the disease and the other of individuals who do not have the disease. The past exposure to the risk factor of the people in both groups is then assessed in some way, for example, by interviewing each person, or by giving each person a questionnaire to complete, or perhaps even seeking the relevant information from friends or relatives of each participant. Once again the results from such a study can be summarized in terms of a 2×2 contingency table as shown in Display 5.4. Note, however, that the table arises in quite a different manner from the corresponding table in a prospective study.

In terms of our investigation of the possible link between excess consumption of chocolate and depression, a retrospective study

The relative risk (RR) is estimated from the 2×2 table shown in Display 5.1.

$$RR = \frac{a/(a+b)}{c/(c+d)}$$

A confidence interval for RR can be constructed from the following formula for the estimation of the standard error of its natural logarithm, $\log_e RR$.

$$s.e.(\log_e RR) = sqrt[1/a - 1/(a+b) + 1/c - 1/(c+d)]$$

Assuming that the distribution of $\log_e RR$ is approximately Normal, a 95% confidence interval for $\log_e RR$ is given by

$$\log_e RR - 1.96 \times s.e.(\log_e RR) \quad to \quad \log_e RR + 1.96 \times s.e.(\log_e RR)$$

In the case of the data in Display 5.2 the relevant calculations are

$$RR = \frac{65/565}{25/675}$$

$$= 3.106$$
$$\log_e(RR) = 1.133$$
$$s.e.(\log_e RR) = sqrt[1/65 - 1/565 + 1/25 - 1/675]$$
$$= 0.228$$

The confidence interval for $\log_e RR$ is, therefore,

$$1.133 - 1.96 \times 0.228 \quad to \quad 1.133 + 1.96 \times 0.228$$

That is,

$$(0.686, 1.589)$$

The final stage is to convert these lower and upper confidence limits to the corresponding limits for RR itself. This is done by simply taking exponents (antilogarithms) of the two limits. The final 95% confidence interval for RR is

$$(e^{0.686}, e^{1.579}) = (1.99, 4.85)$$

DISPLAY 5.3 Estimating relative risk (RR) and its confidence interval

would begin with a group of patients who had been given a diagnosis of depression (the *cases*) and a group who were not depressed (the *controls*) and information collected in some way about their past chocolate-eating habits. A hypothetical set of data is shown in Display 5.5. What can be estimated from these data? Clearly we can calculate exposure rates in each group to give: case exposure

---

(1) Initial stage of a retrospective study (counts)

	Disease present	Disease absent	Total
Risk factor present	unknown	unknown	unknown
Risk factor absent	unknown	unknown	unknown
Total*	$a+c$	$b+d$	$a+b+c+d$

*In terms of the counts subsequently available at the final stage of the study; only the totals $a+b$ and $c+d$ are known since they are fixed by the sampling design.

(2) Final stage of a retrospective study (counts)

	Disease present	Disease absent	Total
Risk factor present	a	b	$a+b$
Risk factor absent	c	d	$c+d$
Total	$a+c$	$b+d$	$a+b+c+d$

(3) Diagrammatic representation of a retrospective study

With disease ——————————————— Exposed / Not exposed

Without disease ——————————————— Exposed / Not exposed

Present —————————————→ Past

Time

DISPLAY 5.4 Retrospective studies

rate = 70/100 (or 70%), control exposure rate = 40/100 (or 40%). But we *cannot* estimate risks in each group as we did in the prospective study, since the number of cases and controls studied is under the control of the investigator and does not reflect the incidence of the disease in the population. By simply changing the number of controls and/or cases, the risks, if estimated as described for the prospective study, could be made to take any value at all! Fortunately if the disease is relatively rare in the population (say below 5%), there is a statistic, known as the **odds ratio**, that acts as an approximation to the relative risk as shown in Display 5.6. The

(1) Initial stage of study (counts)

	Depressed	Not depressed	Total
Chocoholic	unknown	unknown	unknown
Non-chocoholic	unknown	unknown	unknown
Total	100	100	200

(2) Final stage of a prospective study (counts)

	Depressed	Not depressed	Total
Chocoholic	70	40	110
Non-chocoholic	30	60	90
Total	100	100	200

DISPLAY 5.5 Results of a hypothetical retrospective study of the link between consuming large amounts of chocolate and the incidence of depression

estimated odds ratio for the data in Display 5.5 is 3.5. Once again, however, we also need a confidence interval and the relevant calculations are set out in Display 5.7. In this case we see that these calculations lead to an approximate 95% confidence interval of (1.93, 6.36). An odds ratio of one would indicate that there was no association between excessive consumption of chocolate and becoming depressed. Here the confidence interval once again gives evidence that there is a link. (It should be noted that the odds ratio is also often used in prospective studies rather than the relative risk proper.)

One of the major problems in the design of a case-control study is the choice of the appropriate controls. Should they be healthy individuals or patients suffering from an illness unrelated to the one under investigation? With the latter there is always the possibility that the unrelated illness is *also* associated with the supposed risk factor. Smoking cigarettes, for example, appears to increase the risk of several illnesses other than lung cancer.

Even after having decided how to select control subjects, a further decision that must often be made is whether to match each case *individually* with one (or, occasionally, more than one), individual control subject, using characteristics already known (or at least highly likely) to be strongly related to both disease and exposure. Examples of such characteristics might be sex, age, socio-economic

	Disease present	Disease absent	Total
Risk factor present	a	b	a + b
Risk factor absent	c	d	c + d
Total	a + c	b + d	a + b + c + d

Odds in favour of risk factor being present in cases (disease present) = a/c

Odds in favour of risk factor being present in controls (disease absent) = b/d

The odds ratio is

$$OR = \frac{a/c}{b/d} = \frac{ad}{bc}$$

As seen in Display 5.3, relative risk is estimated by

$$RR = \frac{a/(a+b)}{c/(c+d)}$$

If the disease is rare then a will be small relative to b and, similarly, c will be small compared to d. So, $a + b$ can be replaced by a and $c + d$ can be replaced by d in the expression for relative risk, and the result is the odds ratio (approximate relative risk).

DISPLAY 5.6 The odds ratio (OR) as an approximation to relative risk

group etc. This variation of the case-control design can be illustrated by a study reported by Sartwell et al. (1969). The study was conducted in a number of hospitals in several large American cities. In these hospitals all those married women identified as suffering from idiopathic thromboembolism (blood clots) over a three-year period were individually matched with a suitable control. Controls were female patients discharged alive from the same hospital in the same six-month time interval as was the case. In addition, they were individually matched to cases on age, marital status, race, and so on. The history of oral contraceptive use in 175 case-control pairs is summarized in Display 5.8. (Note that although the results can again be arranged in the form of a 2×2 table, it has quite a different structure than those met in the earlier examples. In particular, the entries in each cell now refer to counts of *pairs* of subjects.)

The odds ratio is estimated from the counts in a general 2×2 contingency table by

$$OR = \frac{ad}{bc}$$

A confidence interval for OR can be found from the following formula for the standard error of the natural logarithm of OR

$$\text{s.e.}(\log_e OR) = \text{sqrt}(1/a + 1/b + 1/c + 1/d)$$

Assuming that the sampling distribution of $\log_e OR$ is approximately Normal, a 95% confidence interval for $\log_e OR$ is given by

$$\log_e OR - 1.96 \times \text{s.e.}(\log_e OR) \quad \text{to} \quad \log_e OR + 1.96 \times \text{s.e.}(\log_e OR)$$

Using the example from Display 5.5, the relevant calculations are

$$OR = \frac{70 \times 60}{30 \times 40} = 3.5$$

$$\text{s.e.}(\log_e OR) = \text{sqrt}(1/70 + 1/40 + 1/30 + 1/60)$$
$$= 0.299$$

The confidence interval for $\log_e OR$ is therefore

$$\log_e 3.5 - 1.96 \times 0.299 \quad \text{to} \quad \log_e 3.5 + 1.96 \times 0.299$$

That is:

$$(0.667, 1.839)$$

Once again, the final stage is to take exponents (antilogarithms) of these two limits to find the 95% confidence interval for OR itself. Here they are

$$(e^{0.667}, e^{1.839}) = (1.95, 6.29)$$

DISPLAY 5.7 Estimating the odds ratio (OR) and its confidence interval

From Display 5.8 we see that the proportion of cases who have used oral contraceptives is $(10 + 57)/175$. Similarly, the proportion of controls is $(10 + 13)/175$. Unlike the situation when we are comparing two separate groups of subjects, these two proportions are *not* independent. They are inevitably correlated, because of the 10 pairs who are common to both of the above proportions. Consequently estimation of the odds ratio and a suitable confidence interval have to be modified accordingly. Details are given in

Oral contraceptive use	Number of pairs
Used by both members of the pair	10
Used by the case only	57
Used by the control only	13
Used by neither the case nor the control	95

Tabular (2 × 2) presentation:

		Control		
		User	Non-user	Total
Case	User	$a = 10$	$b = 57$	$a + b = 23$
	Non-user	$c = 13$	$d = 95$	$c + d = 152$
	Total	$a + c = 67$	$b + d = 108$	$a + b + c + d = 175$

DISPLAY 5.8 Past oral contraceptive use in 175 pairs of married women (Sartwell *et al.*, 1969)

Display 5.9. Here these calculations lead to an estimated odds ratio of 4.385 and an approximate 95% confidence interval of (2.40, 8.00). There appears to be a clear link between the use of oral contraceptives and suffering from idiopathic thromboembolism (but see Section 5.3.) (It should be noted that when a variable is used for matching, its role as a possible risk factor *cannot* be investigated, because cases and controls are then automatically similar with respect to that characteristic.)

Confounding variables

Although a high relative risk (or odds ratio) may point towards causation it is almost always possible, as we indicated in the introduction to this chapter, to find alternative explanations for the observed association. In the chocolate and depression study, for example, we have not yet taken into account the gender of the people involved in the study. If we do, suppose the results from our prospective study become as shown in Display 5.10. Now it can be seen that there is no difference between the risk of depression in the male chocoholics and non-chocoholics, and similarly that there is no difference for the corresponding groups of women. The association found in the original data from the prospective study (Display 5.1) where the observations from the two sexes were aggregated is due to the following:

1 Women like to eat chocolate, and
2 Women are more prone to depression.

Here gender is what is known as a *confounding variable* and ignoring it has given rise to a *statistical artefact*. In general, confounding variables are those that are associated both with the risk factor *and* the disease. The worrying conclusion to be gleaned from this less-than-serious example is that there is always a possibility of this type of artefact in epidemiological investigations. One can never be certain that all possible sources of spurious association have been considered and eliminated.

Another problem with epidemiological findings is the determination of the direction of any possible causal links. Even without confounding, the association between chocolate eating and depres-

---

The odds ratio (OR) is now simply estimated as

$$OR = b/c$$

A confidence interval can be constructed from the following formula for the standard error of $\log_e OR$:

$$s.e.(\log_e OR) = sqrt(1/b + 1/c)$$

Assuming approximate Normality for the sampling distribution of $\log_e OR$, a 95% confidence interval for $\log_e OR$ is

$$\log_e OR - 1.96 \times s.e.(\log_e OR) \quad to \quad \log_e OR + 1.96 \times s.e.(\log_e OR)$$

Using the data in Display 5.8,

$$= 57/13 = 4.385$$
$$s.e.(\log_e OR) = sqrt(1/57 + 1/13)$$
$$= 0.307$$

The 95% confidence interval for $\log_e OR$ is

$$\log_e 4.385 - 1.96 \times 0.307 \quad to \quad \log_e 4.385 + 1.96 \times 0.307$$

That is:

$$(0.876, 2.080)$$

The corresponding limits for the confidence interval for OR itself are

$$(e^{0.876}, e^{2.080}) = (2.40, 8.00)$$

DISPLAY 5.9 Estimation of an odds ratio and its confidence interval from a matched pairs case-control study

		Depressed	Not depressed
Men	Chocoholic	5	200
	Non-chocoholic	15	600

Relative risk for men = 1.0

		Depressed	Not depressed
Women	Chocoholic	60	300
	Non-chocoholic	10	50

Relative risk for women = 1.0

*Summing over men and women gives the counts in Display 5.2.

DISPLAY 5.10 Results of a hypothetical prospective study investigating the link between excessive chocolate and depression, in men and women separately*

sion might simply be explained by the fact that depressed people might comfort themselves by eating lots of chocolate!

To illustrate further the problem of confounding variables, a more serious example given by Doll and Hill (1964) will be used. These researchers found a strong association between smoking and subsequent death from alcoholism or cirrhosis of the liver. Six deaths from alcoholism and 27 from cirrhosis of the liver were found amongst those who smoked. No deaths from these causes occurred among non-smokers and the mortality fell almost wholly on the heaviest smokers. But do the observations indicate that smoking causes liver damage? Doll and Hill concluded that this was unlikely, and that a more reasonable explanation of the observed association was that heavy smokers are also often drinkers. Here, alcohol intake is an important confounding variable.

5.3 ADVANTAGES AND DISADVANTAGES OF RETROSPECTIVE AND PROSPECTIVE SURVEYS

Summarizing the previous section, a case-control study involves selecting a sample of patients with a particular disease and comparing their prior exposure to suspected sources of risk with exposure in a comparable control group. The investigation is retrospective and it allows for one to ask about several different suspected risk factors, or even factors associated with *lowering* the incidence of a disease.

The United Kingdom case-control study group (1989) looking primarily at the effect of the use of combined-type oral contraceptives on the incidence of breast cancer, for example, noted also that breast feeding seemed to be associated with a *decreased* risk of breast cancer. It apparently had a protective effect.

A cohort study, on the other hand, involves taking a sample of people thought to be at risk and then comparing their future rates of illness with an appropriate control group who are not thought to be at risk. Here one can investigate the possible associations with the putative risk factor and several different forms of illness. In the classic prospective study of Doll and Hill (1954), for example, the main aim was to try to establish a link between smoking and lung cancer, but they were also able to investigate possible associations between smoking and death due to several other causes.

In general the sequence of investigations in looking for associations between risk factors and diseases, is first to use a retrospective case-control study and if the results are positive, investigate the links further by a prospective study. (A later stage may involve an **intervention trial** to ascertain if modifying the risk factors in patients is followed by a reduction in amount of disease; such trials are discussed in Chapter 6.) In some situations, however, prospective studies are simply impracticable because of the rarity of the illness being investigated.

Case-control studies are simpler and less expensive to carry out than comparable prospective surveys. A prospective study will usually take many years to complete and many subjects might be lost to follow-up or eventually refuse to cooperate with the investigation. There are, however, problems associated with case-control studies. One of these (which has already been mentioned) is the selection of appropriate controls. Another is the selection of entry criteria for the cases themselves. Should they be newly diagnosed patients, for example, or can they include patients with chronic forms of the illness? How homogeneous should the patient group be? Answers to such questions are not necessarily clear-cut, and the reader is referred to Alderson (1983) for a more detailed discussion.

Another source of problems in case-control studies arises from possible recall or response biases. If there is general public concern about a problem (possible associations between childhood leukaemia and proximity to nuclear reactors, for example, or between breast cancer and oral contraceptive use) then the subjects under investigation (particularly if they are one of the cases) are likely to recall or report more events or circumstances thought to have been detrimental to their health than they otherwise might have done. Patients with breast cancer, for example, are quite likely to ruminate over the possible causes of their affliction, including oral contraceptive use. Users of oral contraceptives are likely to be aware of their possible side-effects and suggestions of long-term risks arising from their use. An example of a study in which such an effect may have occurred, is that of Clavel *et al.* (1991). These authors found a small positive association between the use of oral contraceptives and the incidence of breast cancer, but concluded that because the risk did not appear to change with duration of use, age at first use or change of brand, it might be an effect of information bias arising from the widespread attention given to the problem. One way of reducing bias is through not letting the subjects or the interviewer(s) know the real reason for the study. One might also ensure that the interviewer is 'blind' by not revealing whether the subject is a case or a control.

The information collected in a prospective study is likely to be less subject to bias than that obtained from a retrospective one. Nevertheless, subtle biases are still a possibility. Alderson (1983), for example, considers studies designed to investigate association between diet and heart disease. Case-control studies are suspect because the collection of dietary histories is of questionable validity, and the actual occurrence of heart disease may have affected the subjects' appetite and attitude to diet. One would, therefore, conclude that a prospective study would be a better bet. One simply collects dietary information in a sample of healthy subjects and monitors both their diet and patterns of sickness and health over time. The problem arises, however, that this monitoring itself might affect a subject's eating habits and other aspects of his or her lifestyle.

FURTHER READING

Abramson, J.H. (1988). *Making sense of data: a self-instructional manual on the interpretation of epidemiological data*. Oxford: Oxford University Press. Section D (Making sense of associations).

Gardner, M.J. and Altman, D.G. (1989). *Statistics with confidence*. London: British Medical Journal. (Chapter 6.)

EXERCISES

1 In a retrospective study concerned with assessing whether the amount of pre-natal care received by a pregnant woman affected the risk that her child died, data were collected from two clinics. Amount of care was categorized into 'more than normal' and 'less than normal'. The results are shown in the table below:

	Infant's survival			
	Died		Survived	
Amount of care:	*Less*	*More*	*Less*	*More*
Clinic A	3	4	176	293
Place of care				
Clinic B	17	2	197	23

(a) Calculate the 95% confidence interval for the odds ratio in each clinic. What do you conclude from these intervals?

(b) Combine the data over clinics and calculate the odds ratio for the aggregated data. What would your conclusion be based solely on the evidence of the aggregated data?

(c) Explain the difference between the results of (a) and (b).

2 Adelusi (1977) reported the results of a case-control study designed to investigate whether control characteristics are associated with the subsequent development of cervical cancer. The cases were married Nigerian women with a histologic diagnosis of invasive cancer of the cervix. The control group consisted of healthy married women of child-bearing age. A questionnaire was administered to each woman, on which they were asked about their sexual habits, in particular the age at which they first had sexual intercourse. The results are shown below:

Age at first coitus	Cases	Controls
≤15 years	36	78
>15 years	11	95
Total	47	173

Calculate a 95% confidence interval for the odds ratio. Does age at first coitus appear to be a risk factor for the development of cervical cancer?

3 Janerich *et al.* (1980) compared oral contraceptive usage among mothers of malformed infants and matched controls who give

birth to healthy children. The controls were matched for maternal age and race of mother. The table below shows the counts of women who conceived while using the pill or immediately following use

| | | **Case** | |
		Yes	No
	Yes	1	33
Control			
	No	49	632

Calculate the odds ratio and a 99% confidence interval. What conclusions might you draw from the result?

Treatment Trials

6.1 INTRODUCTION

If a doctor claims that a certain type of psychotherapy will cure patients of their depression, or that vitamin C prevents or cures the common cold, how do we assess these claims? How do we know if AZT is likely to help prevent the development of AIDS or that radiotherapy will prevent the recurrence of breast cancer? What sort of evidence do we need to decide that claims about the efficacy of clinical treatments are, indeed, valid? One thing is certain: we should not rely on the views of experts, unless these views are backed by sound empirical evidence. Ideally such evidence should be collected in a way that makes the interpretation of the data unequivocal so that finally we are able to say 'Patients receiving Treatment X get better (or do not, as the case may be) and that the patients are getting better *as a direct result of receiving Treatment X.*' Typically, we are likely to be more concerned with a **comparative** statement of the type 'Patients receiving Treatment X do better (or worse) than those receiving Treatment Y, and this is solely attributable to the treatment differences.' Given these aims it would clearly be of little use, in a comparative experiment, giving Treatment X, for example, only to female patients and Treatment Y only to the males. There would always be the risk in that case that any treatment differences observed (or not observed) might be due to confounding differences between the sexes. Similarly, it would be unwise to rely on differences between the outcomes for patients receiving Treatment X *now* with those who have received an older treatment, Y, at some time in the past, since again there might be confounding differences between the present group of patients and those treated in the past. So, how should we go about collecting valid empirical data to assess possible treatment effects?

There is clearly a need for some form of carefully controlled experiment for uncovering the relative effects of differing treatments (these 'treatments' including doing nothing or giving the patient an inert tablet called a placebo). Such a need has been met by the development of the **controlled randomized clinical trial**.

6.2 THE DESIGN OF CLINICAL TRIALS

A clinical trial may be defined as a medical experiment designed to evaluate which (if any) of two or more treatments is the more effective. Effectiveness can be measured in terms of disappearance of symptoms, a drop in symptom severity, quicker recovery, the prevention of recurrence of symptoms or of the initial development of symptoms (as in the development of full-blown AIDS in HIV-infected individuals, for instance), and so on. Ideally we might be concerned with cures, but almost as important is the ability to control symptom severity, to slow down the progress of a chronically debilitating or fatal illness, or to improve the quality of life of say, a permanently handicapped patient. To reiterate the point made in the Introduction, the fundamental reason for a clinical trial is **comparison**, and in order to make a comparison, we need control groups. The control patients will vary depending on the purpose of the trial. If there is no treatment that has already been demonstrated to be effective then it would be reasonable to test a new drug, for example, against a placebo. If there is already a well-established treatment that is *known* to be effective (from the results of previous controlled trials) then it would be much more sensible to compare the effects of the new treatment with those in a control group treated with the well-established method. Whatever is chosen as the appropriate control, we then need a mechanism of allocating the competing treatments. At the end of the trial we need to be able to say with considerable confidence that any differences that have been observed have arisen solely because of differences between the treatments.

So how should patients be allocated to the competing treatment groups in a trial? Perhaps the clinician should decide? Possibly, but then the results of the trial would be viewed with a considerable amount of scepticism! The clinician might, for example, allocate the patients with the worst prognosis to the promising new therapy and the better ones to the older one (no doubt with the best possible intention in respect of her patients). Or older patients might receive the traditional therapy and youngsters the new one, and so on. All of these procedures would tend to invalidate any resulting findings. Should the patients themselves decide what treatment they receive? Again this would be highly undesirable. They are likely to believe that the new therapy is about to solve all of their problems. Why else would it be featuring in the trial? What patient would knowingly choose a placebo? So perhaps the first patients to volunteer to take part in the trial should all be given the novel treatment, for example, and the later ones used as controls? Again, early volunteers might be the more seriously ill patients, those desperate to find a new remedy that works.

In a modern controlled trial none of the ad hoc allocation procedures considered above (or others not described), would be regarded as satisfactory. Instead, the treatment to be given to each individual patient is decided by chance: by *random allocation*. One could simply flip a coin each time a patient enters the trial and allocate the patient to the new treatment if the result is 'heads', or to the control group otherwise, although a more sophisticated randomization procedure is generally used in a real trial. The essential feature is, however, the role of randomization rather than the mechanism used to achieve it.

The role of randomization

Randomization serves several purposes. First, it provides an impartial method for the allocation of treatment to the patients, free from personal biases. This means that treatment comparisons will not be invalidated by the way in which the clinician, for example, might choose to allocate treatments if left to use his or her judgement. Even if there was no intention to bias the results, the clinician might inadvertently allocate the patients with the most severe symptoms to the new treatment, or vice versa. This may not happen of course but, to convince a sceptical observer, it is better to ensure that the design precludes any such possibility. The second, and major, advantage of randomization is that it tends to balance treatment groups in respect of the effects of extraneous factors that may influence the outcome of treatment. Randomization distributes these influences by chance so that on average (over repeated trials) there will be no advantage of one treatment group over another because of the way in which the treatments have been allocated. That is, random allocation removes the possibility of allocation biases. It might be thought that this problem could also be overcome by making an effort to identify what extraneous variables (sex, age, severity, and so on) might influence the outcome of treatment. One could then ensure that there is no bias introduced by balancing the numbers of patients of the different types within the treatment groups exactly (that is, by ensuring that there are exactly the same number of men, for example, receiving each of the treatments). Unfortunately there is no way of knowing if we have overlooked an important extraneous variable. Randomization, however, offers control over possible biases of this type, even in respect of those confounding factors not suspected of being a problem. Randomization does not guarantee that treatment groups will be exactly comparable in any given trial but it does ensure that, on average, there will be comparability. Furthermore, it enables us to determine valid confidence intervals for treatment effects (differences), taking into account chance fluctuations one would expect to result from the random allocation procedure. If allocation were to be decided by a subjective mechanism, even though in an apparently haphazard manner, this would undermine the validity of the resulting confidence intervals as well as leading to questions about potential bias.

Blinding

Having allocated patients to their respective treatments it is vital that they are then treated in exactly the same way, except with respect to that aspect of their therapy being tested. If the patients receiving a new drug treatment were monitored much more closely than the controls, or received more counselling and support, then any resulting 'treatment' differences might really be due to the different monitoring procedures adopted. One way of ensuring comparability of the different arms of a trial is to make sure that no one involved in the patient's care knows to which of the competing treatments the patient has actually been allocated. In this case the treating clinician(s) and support staff are ignorant in respect of the treatment allocation, as are the patient and anyone assessing the outcome of the treatment. Such an arrangement is known as a **double-blind** trial. In the case of an oral drug therapy, for example, the competing tablets can be made to look and taste just the same. Alternatively, it is possible to manufacture a placebo tablet which is in every way identical to the active one, except that it does not contain the active ingredient under test.

In many cases, however, it is clearly impracticable or unethical to run a double-blind trial. How could a surgeon be blind to the surgical procedure being used on a given patient? A surgical patient might possibly be blind but the procedures required ensure this blindness would usually be unacceptable. Pocock (1983), for example, points out that it would clearly be unacceptable to subject a control group to an incision under anaesthetic to mimic genuine surgery. Having said this, however, psychiatrists have evaluated electro-convulsive therapy in the treatment of depression by treating the patients in both arms of a trial in exactly the same way (including the use of the now customary anaesthesia), except that the treated group actually received the electric shock and the controls did not (no current was delivered)—see Johnstone et al. (1980).

In cases where double-blind trials are not possible, potential biases in treatment comparisons can be lessened, or even removed entirely, by arranging for the assessment and evaluation of outcome to be carried out blind, that is with the assessor being unaware of which treatment each patient received.

Historical controls

Despite overwhelming support from statisticians for the idea that patients should be randomly assigned to one or other form of treatment, it is not intuitively appealing to many in the medical profession or indeed to many laymen. The reasons are not difficult to identify. The clinician faced with the responsibility of restoring the patient to health and suspecting that any new treatment is likely to have advantages over the old, may be unhappy that many patients will be receiving, in her view, the less valuable treatment. (The clinician is aware that the new treatment is unproven—otherwise there would be no need for a trial. But she is worried by the thought that there must be *some* basis for its effectiveness, whether it be *in vitro*, in animals or on a small scale in patients.) Likewise the patient being recruited for such a trial and having been made aware of the randomization component, might be troubled by the possibility of receiving an 'inferior' treatment. The extent of this ethical problem will depend largely on what is at stake. In trials of a new compound to alleviate backache it is unlikely to be of the same degree of concern as in trials of a possible cure for patients with AIDS. (The ethical issues involved with clinical trials are discussed in more detail in the next section.)

Because of such fears, alternatives to random allocation have been sought, and one which avoids randomization altogether is the use of ***historical controls***. With this approach, *all* suitable patients receive the new treatment and their responses and outcomes are compared with those obtained from the records of patients previously given the old treatment. Such a procedure overcomes the ethical dilemma described above, but unfortunately it has a major difficulty associated with it. The use of historical controls presupposes that everything *except the new treatment being investigated*, has remained constant in time. The type of patient, the severity of the illness, the ancillary treatment given, the measurements made, *all* must be equivalent for the previously treated patients as those currently receiving the new treatment for it to be appropriate to conclude that any apparent improvement in patient response is truly due to this treatment. Unfortunately, it is very unlikely that all the conditions indicated above will have remained the same. Past observations, for example, are unlikely to relate to a precisely similar group of patients. The quality of the information collected on historical controls will almost certainly be inferior to that extracted from the current patients, since it would have arisen only in the context of routine clinical practice rather than as a result of a special investigation. Patients being given a new, and as yet, unproven treatment are likely to be far more closely monitored and receive more intensive ancillary care than historical controls receiving the orthodox treatment and not in a trial. Patients on a new therapy who fare badly may be excluded from the final analysis, whereas the corresponding exclusion of any historical controls is difficult since considerable time will have elapsed since they were treated.

Because of such problems, trials which use historical controls are far more likely to *overestimate* the efficacy of a new treatment, than the corresponding randomized trial. Apart from the obvious disadvantages of such spurious findings, they may also make it more difficult to arrange for a properly conducted randomized trial to be performed, since many clinicians, having seen the results from a historical control trial may be reluctant to randomize patients to a treatment that they now consider inferior. An illustration of the possible bias produced by historical control trials is provided by the results shown in Display 6.1, taken from Sacks *et al.* (1983). The historical control trials show a preponderance of results in which the new treatment is shown to be effective. This bias, in favour of the new therapy, is a general feature of historical control trials.

Therapy	Randomized trials		Historical control trials	
	new treatment effective	new treatment not effective	new treatment effective	new treatment not effective
Coronary artery surgery	1	7	16	5
Anticoagulants for acute myocardial infarction	1	9	5	1
Surgery for oesophageal varices	0	8	4	1
Fluorouracil for colon cancer	0	5	2	0
BCG immunotherapy for melanoma	2	2	4	0
Diethylstilbestrol for habitual abortion	0	3	5	0

DISPLAY 6.1 Published clinical trials for six medical areas (Sacks *et al.*, 1983)

Historical control trials become less objectionable when the results from the new treatment are compared with results of recent studies with the older treatment, that have involved similar kinds of patients and similar criteria for evaluating response. But even here Byar *et al.* (1976) suggest that there is limited protection against bias introduced by time changes in the nature of the patient population or in supportive care and diagnostic criteria. (Some arguments in favour of carefully constructed historical control trials are given in Gehan and Freireich (1974) and Gehan (1983). In addition, Pocock (1983), suggests that the case for such trials becomes more convincing in situations where there are very limited numbers of patients available for a randomized trial.)

Ethics of trial design

Perhaps the most serious objections to randomized clinical trials involve ethical issues, and despite their increasing acceptance, there is still concern amongst many clinicians that randomized trials can violate the doctor–patient relationships. Part of the difficulty according to Byar *et al.* (1976), arises in defining in a manner agreeable to everyone what constitutes ethical behaviour. This is clearly a problem, but in the main the ethical dilemma involves the conflict between trying to ensure that each individual patient receives the treatment most beneficial for his or her condition, and evaluating competing therapies as efficiently as possible, so that all future patients might benefit from the superior treatment. Lellouch and Schwartz (1971) refer to the problem as competition between *individual* and *collective* ethics. Pocock (1983) suggests that each clinical trial requires a balance between the two: the prime motivation for conducting a trial involves collective ethics, but individual ethics have to be given as much attention as possible without destroying the trial's validity. A further very important point made by Pocock is that it is unethical to conduct trials which are of such poor quality that they cannot make a meaningful contribution to medical knowledge.

These points have a number of implications for clinicians considering taking part in a randomized controlled trial, which are nicely summarized in the following two quotations from Shaw and Chalmers (1970).

(a) Patients should not be admitted who could not be assigned without hesitation to any of the study therapies by all of the participating physicians. For one physician to admit patients that another would reject is ethically inappropriate and scientifically undesirable.

(b) Assume that several physicians believe that a scientific clinical trial is needed and is ethical ... what should the physician who rather reluctantly agrees that *perhaps* a trial is desirable, do? Such a physician should stay out of the study unless he can faithfully and in good conscience follow without bias the specific rules of the study. A physician's behaviour is both unethical and unscientific if he joins a study and then begins to undermine its soundness by biased actions.

Even in situations in which there are no ethical problems in beginning a randomized clinical trial, such problems may arise for a variety of reasons during the course of a trial. One which is relatively simple to deal with is when a patient's condition seems to be deteriorating; here the ethical obligation must always and entirely outweigh any experimental considerations. This obligation means that whenever a physician thinks that the interests of her patient are at stake, she must be free to treat the patient as she sees fit. This is an absolutely essential requirement for an ethically conducted trial, no matter what complications it may introduce into the final analysis of the data. (A well-designed trial will try to make clear the conditions under which a patient should be withdrawn from the trial, before the trial begins.)

According to Bracken (1987) many clinician's ethical problems with clinical trials would be eased if they could accept their uncertainty about much of what they practise. Bracken suggests that when doctors *are* able to admit to themselves and their patients uncertainty about the best action to take, then no conflict exists between the roles of the doctor and the scientist. He concludes that in such circumstances it cannot be less ethical to choose a treatment by random allocation within a controlled trial, than to choose what happens to be readily available, by hunch, or what a drug company recommends. Perhaps the most effective argument in favour of randomized clinical trials is that the alternative, practising in complacent uncertainty, is worse.

6.3 EXAMPLES OF CLINICAL TRIALS

Clinical trials are of considerable importance in modern medical research, and over the last four decades or so they have been used to evaluate a vast array of new drugs and treatment. But as pointed out by Hill (1962), they are, in principal at least, far from new, and it is worthwhile considering the following account of an eighteenth-century 'trial' described by Lind (1753).

On the 20th May, 1747, I took twelve patients in the scurvy, on board the Salisbury at sea. Their cases were as similar as I could have them. They all in general had putrid gums, the spots and lassitude, with weakness of their knees. They lay together in one place, being a proper apartment for the sick the fore-hold; and had one diet in common to all, viz. water-gruel sweetened with sugar in the morning, fresh mutton broth often times for dinner; at other times puddings, boiled biscuit with sugar etc. And for supper, barley and raisins, rice and currants, sago and wine, or the like. Two of these were ordered each a quart of cider a day. Two others took twenty-five gutts of elixir vitriol three times a day, upon an empty stomach; using a gargle strongly acidulated with it for their mouths. Two others took two spoonfuls of vinegar three times a day, upon an empty stomach; having their gruels and their other food well acidulated with it, as also the gargle for their mouths. Two of the worst patients, with the tendons in the ham rigid (a symptom none of the rest had) were put under a course of sea-water. Of this they drank half a pint every day; and sometimes more or less as it operated, by way of a gentle physic. Two others had each two oranges and one lemon given them every day. These they eat with greediness at different times, upon an empty stomach. They continued but six days under this course, having consumed the quantity that could be spared. The two remaining patients, took the bigness of a nutmeg three times a day of an electuary recommended by a hospital-surgeon, made of garlic, mustard-feed, rad.raphan, balsam of Peru, and gum myrr; using for common drink barley water well acidulated with tamarinds; by a decoction of which, with the addition of cremor tartar, they were greatly purged three or four times during the course.

The consequence was, that the most sudden and visible good effects were perceived from the use of the oranges and lemons; one of those who had taken them, being at the end of six days fit for duty. The spots were not indeed at that time quite off his body, nor his gums sound; but without any other medicine, than a gargle of elixir vitriol, he became quite healthy before we came into Plymouth, which was on the 16th June. The other was the best recovered of any in his condition; and being now deemed pretty well, was appointed nurse to the rest of the sick.

Lind's experiment contains two essentials of a well-conducted trial. The first is that groups of patients subjected to different treatments are compared. The second is that there is well defined means of assessing outcome. Perhaps Lind did not use randomization to form his treatment groups but in many other respects his investigation is similar to a modern clinical trial.

Salk polio vaccine trial

The first outbreak of poliomyelitis did not occur until 1916. By the 1950s thousands of Americans, particularly children, had contracted the disease, with devastating effects on their lives. Several vaccines had been developed, but that of Dr J. Salk was chosen for a large-scale trial, on the basis that it had proved successful at generating antibodies to polio during laboratory tests. Since the annual incidence rate of polio was only about 1 in 2000, several thousand subjects had to be recruited and the study was on a massive scale with a large staff.

Given the nature of the disease there were, not surprisingly, objections to the use of a placebo-treated control group. These were overcome, however, on the grounds that polio tends to occur in the form of an epidemic. Consequently if an uncontrolled study had found a drop in 1954 compared to previous years it may simply have been due to a natural short-term decline in the disease. So the investigation whilst large, was, in essence, quite simple; properly randomized subjects were allocated to two treatments and all inoculated before the polio season began. The study was double blind, using saline fluid injections for the control group to mimic the active vaccinations. There was some problem with regard to what should be used as the outcome measure—deaths, paralytic disease or all confirmed diagnoses—but, fortunately the results were decisive *whatever* count was used as shown in Display 6.2 (taken from Meier, 1975).

Vitamin C and the common cold

In his book, *Vitamin C and the common cold*, Linus Pauling claimed that ascorbic acid (Vitamin C), in large daily doses could prevent upper respiratory infections. As a prophylactic measure he recommended 1 to 3 g daily. Pauling's advice was based on a combination of the results from a number of clinical trials, personal experience and evolutionary considerations. A trial which appears to give some support to Dr Pauling's ideas is that reported in Coulehan *et al.* (1974). Children in a boarding school were randomly allocated to receive either daily Vitamin C or a placebo, and were observed over a 14-week period. Several measures of outcome were used but one analysis involved children who remained well throughout the study as contrasted with those having at least one day sick. The results are shown in Display 6.3. The calculated odds ratios and their associated confidence intervals demonstrate that, with the exception of upper-grade boys, the odds in favour of no sickness days is greater in the group treated with vitamin C.

A further trial of ascorbic acid for the common cold is reported by Lewis *et al.* (1975). In this trial 311 people were randomly assigned to four groups. Group one received placebo both for maintenance *and* for therapy when they contracted a cold. Group two received

Illness rate per 100 000 (number of cases)			
	Vaccinated		*Placebo*
All reported	40.8	(82)	80.5 (162)
Confirmed polio	28.4	(57)	70.6 (142)
Paralytic polio	16.4	(33)	57.1 (115)
Fatal polio	—	(0)	— (2)
Number inoculated	200,745		201,229

DISPLAY 6.2 Results of the Salk polio vaccine trial (Meier, 1975)

Lower grade

Male

	Children who were never ill	Children ill at least 1 day	Total
Vitamin C	31	50	81
Placebo	18	69	87

Estimated odds ratio   2.38
95% confidence interval   (1.20, 4.72)

Female

	Children who were never ill	Children ill at least 1 day	Total
Vitamin C	30	79	109
Placebo	12	93	105

Estimated odds ratio   2.94
95% confidence interval   (1.41, 6.13)

Upper grade

Male

	Children who were never ill	Children ill at least 1 day	Total
Vitamin C	40	22	62
Placebo	34	27	61

Estimated odds ratio   1.44
95% confidence interval   (0.70, 2.98)

Female

	Children who were never ill	Children ill at least 1 day	Total
Vitamin C	42	27	69
Placebo	29	38	67

Estimated odds ratio   2.04
95% confidence interval   (1.03, 4.04)

DISPLAY 6.3 Comparison of children on vitamin C or placebo: whether ill during active surveillance (Coulehan *et al.*, 1974)

placebo maintenance but ascorbic acid for colds. Group three received ascorbic acid maintenance and placebo for colds, and Group four received ascorbic acid for both maintenance and therapy. The study continued for a 9-month period. Outcome measures included number of colds per person, mean duration of colds and time at home. Display 6.4 shows the number of people completing the study and the average number of colds per person for each of the four treatment groups. The cold duration averaged 7.1 days for the placebo group, 6.6 days for those taking 3g of Vitamin C per day either as maintenance or placebo, and 5.9 days for those in the 6g Vitamin C group. The authors concluded that the Vitamin C treatment might shorten colds to a small degree.

AIDS and AZT

One of the most disturbing developments in medicine during the last part of the twentieth century has been the rapid and continuing rise, particularly in some parts of the world, of the incidence of AIDS, the acquired immunodeficiency syndrome. AIDS is characterized by severe immunodeficiency, life-threatening opportunistic infections, neoplasia and a fatal outcome. The underlying immune defect in AIDS is caused by infection with a human retrovirus, HIV. Since the early 1980s, the search for treatments that might combat AIDS has been undertaken by numerous research groups. One such group (Mitsuya *et al.*, 1985) discovered that the drug azidothymidine (AZT) inhibited HIV replication *in vitro*. Consequently it was considered appropriate that the drug should be subjected to a trial on patients suffering from AIDS. A double-blind, placebo-controlled trial was instigated by Fischl *et al.* (1987). Of 282 patients with AIDS recruited into the trial, 145 received AZT and 137 received placebo. During the 24 weeks of the study, 19 placebo recipients and a single AZT recipient died. The estimated odds ratio is 0.043 with a 95% confidence interval of (0.001, 0.28). Not surprisingly the researchers concluded that their data demonstrated that AZT administration decreased mortality in patients with

Group			
Prophylactic	Therapeutic	Number of patients	Mean duration (days)
Placebo	Placebo	65	7.1
Placebo	Vitamin C	56	6.5
Vitamin C	Placebo	52	6.7
Vitamin C	Vitamin C	76	5.9

DISPLAY 6.4 Mean duration of colds in a vitamin C trial (Lewis *et al.*, 1975)

AIDS. But unfortunately, as always, life was not really so straight-forward! In another trial of AZT (Richman *et al.*, 1987), serious adverse reactions were found amongst the AZT users, particularly bone marrow suppression. In addition patients in the AZT group reported more myalgia and nausea (see Display 6.5). Secondly, doubts were shed on the validity of earlier trial results because treatment groups unblinded themselves in the first few weeks, which could have resulted in bias. Lastly some researchers even suggested that AZT may not exert a specifically antiviral action.

The whole issue of treatment of AIDS with AZT continues to be extremely controversial and highlights the great difficulties of running a properly randomized, controlled trial for a disease which is ultimately always fatal. When the initial placebo controlled trial was planned, a number of organizations were highly critical that some patients would not receive AZT treatment, and pressure from these organizations led to the rapid approval of the drug by the United States of America regulatory body, the Food and Drug Administration (FDA). With the identification of the serious side-

Adverse reaction	AZT group (N = 145)	Placebo group (N = 137)	Odds ratio: Approx. 95% C.I.*
Anorexia	16	11	(0.63, 3.18)
Asthenia	27	25	(0.56, 1.87)
Diarrhoea	18	25	(0.33, 1.22)
Dizziness	8	6	(0.43, 1.77)
Fever	23	16	(0.72, 2.83)
Headache	61	51	(0.76, 1.98)
Insomnia	7	1	(0.84, 56.85)
Malaise	11	9	(0.47, 2.91)
Myalgia	11	3	(1.00, 13.44)
Nausea	66	25	(2.17, 6.44)
Pain in abdomen	25	20	(0.64, 2.31)
	0	4	—
Photosensitivity	24	21	(0.58, 2.07)
Rash	11	12	(0.36, 2.01)
Somnolence	7	11	(0.22, 1.54)
Taste perversion			

*Based on exponent of log $\pm$ 1.96 standard errors

DISPLAY 6.5 Number of patients reporting adverse reactions in an AZT trial (Fischl *et al.*, 1987)

effects associated with using AZT, and the growing doubts about its efficacy, the same organizations changed their attitude to the drug to the extent of campaigning against its more widespread prescription. Help groups were even established to enable HIV-positive patients gain the confidence to come off their medication!

6.4 TRIAL SIZE AND META ANALYSIS

One of the most frequent questions faced by the statistician acting as adviser to medical researchers is 'How many patients do I need?' Whatever type of statistical design is used for a study, this question of sample size is fundamental. Practical, ethical and statistical issues are all involved in determining the sample size needed for an investigation. Considering first the ethical issues, a study with too many subjects may be deemed unethical through the unnecessary involvement of extra people. Such studies are rare! On the other hand, studies with samples that are too small will be unlikely to detect clinically important effects. Such investigations are also usually regarded as unethical in their use of patients and other resources. Studies which are too small and which lack statistical power are, unfortunately, only too common. It is increasingly recognized, however, that few studies can involve sufficient patients to resolve, once and for all, important clinical questions. It is more likely that many small or medium-sized trials will be carried out, with the hope that the results may eventually be *combined* in some way to give an overall answer to the particular question of interest. The term *meta analysis* has been used to describe the process of evaluating and combining the results of existing clinical trials.

Meta analysis

Sometimes called *overviewing* or *pooling*, meta analysis refers to a collection of techniques whereby the results of two or more independent studies are statistically combined to yield an overall answer to a question of interest. The method has become increasingly popular over the last decade. Examples include combining results from studies of beta-blockers in post myocardial infarction (Yusuf *et al.*, 1985), aspirin in coronary heart disease (Breddin *et al.*, 1979) and antibiotic prophylaxis in colon surgery (Baum *et al.*, 1981). Full details of the statistical bases of meta analysis in given in Fleiss (1993). Here we consider briefly one example of its use and some of its problems.

Acupuncture is increasingly used by the general public to alleviate conditions as varied as asthma, back strain, tennis elbow and migraine. Its clinical efficiency remains unproven, however, since the trials in which the procedure has been investigated have, individually, been inconclusive. Consequently, Patel *et al.* (1989) undertook a meta analysis of all trials of acupuncture for treatment of chronic pain published in English, from 1970 onwards, that met particular selection criteria. The results for 14 trials were summarized in terms of confidence intervals for relative risk estimated from the proportions of patients improving etc. Display 6.6 graphs these confidence intervals. Only two of the 14 trials obtained the result that patients treated with acupuncture did worse, on average, than the control group. The 95% confidence intervals for four of these 14 trials did not include the 'zero risk difference' result. All four favoured acupuncture.

Meta analysis is not without its critics, Oakes (1986, 1993) is particularly sceptical, and it is clear that many problems need to be confronted if such an approach is to lead to sensible and acceptable conclusions. A fundamental question that confronts anyone who

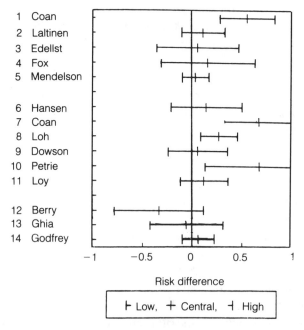

DISPLAY 6.6 Confidence intervals for relative risk from acupuncture trials (reproduced from Patel *et al.*, 1989)

wishes to summarize a body of research is 'What studies should be included?' Should only randomized trials be included? Should poor-quality research be excluded (and who should judge)? Peto (1987) for example, suggests that only randomized trials be considered. Many meta analysts would probably want to exclude studies which they thought were of poor quality. Fleiss (1987) takes a different view, however, arguing that such studies *should* be included since judgements about how serious a study is flawed are likely to be very subjective.

A further question posed by Oakes is 'To what population does the inference or estimate resulting from meta analysis apply?' When the trials included have sufficient similarity of patients then the answer is likely to be relatively clear. In some cases however, the combination of studies involving very different types of patients will make the question far more taxing. In a pooled analysis of the use of steroids for peptic ulcer disease, for example, one study combined 16 trials involving children with 55 studies involving adults! A detailed account of the problem of meta analysis is given in Begg and Berlin (1988).

6.5 SOME PROBLEMS OF CLINICAL TRIALS

The design and analysis of clinical trials often involves a number of difficult issues and problems. A detailed account of many of these is given in Pocock (1983). Here we will briefly consider some of the most important.

Intention-to-treat analysis

A complication that arises in many trials is that of patients who fail to complete the intended course of treatment and who are either removed from the trial or, in some cases, switched to the alternative therapy group or a therapy different from any prescribed in the protocol. Display 6.7 shows a diagrammatic representation of the possibilities.

Statistically the appropriate way of dealing with the observation arising from such a trial is by ***intention-to-treat analysis***. Essentially this means that all patients randomly allocated to one of the treatments in a trial should be analysed together as representing that treatment, whether or not they completed, or even received the

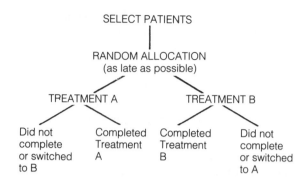

DISPLAY 6.7 A simplified schema for a randomized clinical trial (reproduced with permission from Newell 1992)

treatment. In intention-to-treat analysis, the randomization not only decides the treatment allocation, it decides there and then how the patient's data will be analysed, whether or not the patient actually receives the prescribed treatment.

Analysis based on intention-to-treat may appear to offend intuition and clinicians may often press for comparisons based on the treatment actually received rather than the treatment prescribed. There are, however, several arguments against this approach. First, the balance of extraneous variables brought about by randomization is likely to be disturbed, causing the validity of the statistical procedures to be undermined. Second, results of analysis by treatment received may suffer from a bias introduced by using compliance, a factor often related to outcome, to determine the groups for comparison.

Excellent accounts of the intention-to-treat principle, which include a number of examples of what can go wrong if the principle is ignored, are given in Newell (1992) and Peduzzi *et al.* (1991).

Incomplete follow up—drop-outs

One of the most difficult problems facing the researcher analysing a longitudinal clinical trial is what to do about patients who simply disappear from the trial all together or fail to appear for one of their scheduled visits? Heyting *et al.* (1992) list the common causes of patients prematurely ceasing to participate. They are

- Recovery
- Lack of improvement

- Unwanted signs or symptoms that may be related to the investigational treatment
- Unpleasant study procedures
- Concurrent health problems
- External reasons that seem to be unrelated to the trial procedures or to the progress of the patient.

These causes may operate singly or in combination. The initiative to end participation may be taken by the patient, by the physician or jointly. It is easy to appreciate that such a variety of possible causes for drop-outs is likely to complicate the statistical analysis of such data.

It might seem that the simplest procedure for dealing with drop-outs, at least if there are not too many of them, would be to simply exclude them from the analysis. Heyting *et al.* (1992), however, give some illustrations of the serious bias that can result from this approach. Suppose, for example, that treatment A is modestly effective in a proportion of the patients, regardless of the initial severity of their illness, while treatment B causes the less severely ill patients to recover and leaves the severely ill patients essentially unaffected. If the recovered patients tended to drop out before the final assessment time, a simple-minded comparison of an outcome measure of illness severity for those patients completing the study will unduly favour treatment A. The bias would be accentuated if treatment A caused some of the treatment-resistant patients to drop out due to the unfavourable balance between side-effects and improvement in the severity of their illness.

If only one or two patients drop out of the trial then any biases introduced by leaving them out of the analysis are likely to be small. In many trials, however, other procedures for handling drop-outs need to be considered. Many have been suggested and details are given in Everitt (1994).

Interim analyses

In many clinical trials patients are entered one at a time and their responses to treatment observed sequentially. As data accumulates, investigators may use it to check, amongst other things, protocol compliance and the incidence of adverse side-effects. Such checks are clearly sensible and non-contentious. Interim analysis are, however, most often used to look for treatment differences which are large and convincing enough to terminate or change the trial at a stage earlier than originally planned. The rationale of this being to ensure that the maximum number of patients receive the most effective course of treatment. Whilst it is obviously ethically desirable to terminate a clinical trial early if one therapy is clearly better than the alternative being tested, interim analyses are rarely straightforward and often raise difficult statistical problems. It is not appropriate to discuss these here but details are given in Everitt (1994).

6.6 READING A CLINICAL TRIAL REPORT

In this section we will simply pose a series of questions (the answers will usually be found elsewhere in the chapter).

- Was the allocation of patients to treatments randomized? If not, how were the treatments allocated? It is not always possible to allocate individual patients in a trial randomly, although this is routinely expected in drugs trials. If one wished to evaluate the performance of a new clinical service, for example, a randomized experiment might be precluded for practical reasons. If randomization was not used, how do the authors justify their allocation procedure, and are you convinced by their arguments?
- Apart from the randomization itself, what are the other features of the trials design? Did the authors allocate patients to two independent groups, for example, or did they match pairs of similar patients and then randomly allocate one of each pair to the new treatment? Such changes in design have implications for the subsequent analysis of the results. Do the authors acknowledge this? Does the report show evidence of an appropriate form of statistical analysis? We are aware that the answers about the technicalities concerning the link between esoteric designs and the appropriate form of statistical inference are beyond the scope of the present text. If, however, the authors describe a rather complex or unusual trial design and then do not make any effort to describe how the design was allowed for in the analysis, you might be justified in suspecting that something is wrong.
- Were the results for *all* of the patients who were allocated to treatment entered into the estimation of treatment effects? If not, why not? Were there many drop-outs, and do the authors discuss the reasons for drop out and evaluate their effect on the results? In the estimation of treatment effects, were all the

patients kept in the groups to which they were randomly allocated, rather than in those to which they had subsequently drifted?

- Who was blind? In particular, were the assessors of treatment outcome blind? If not, why not? Do the authors discuss how problems of blindness (or more appropriately, lack of it) might have biased the results?
- Did the patients all get comparable treatment, apart from that aspect of the treatment under test? Were the treatment groups similar at the beginning of the trial? Did the authors allow for known prognostic factors in the analysis of the trial results? Although random allocation would have allowed for possible biases due to lack of balance in these prognostic factors, an appropriate statistical analysis in which prognostic factors are allowed for can still improve the precision of the estimates of the treatment effects. Again, this is beyond the scope of this book.
- How large were the differences between treatments? What was the precision of the estimates? That is, what were the appropriate confidence intervals? Is the lack of precision, if present, likely to be the result of inadequate numbers of patients entering the trial? Do the authors appear to distinguish between statistical and clinical importance?

6.7 SUMMARY

Many statisticians regard the controlled clinical trial as one of their greatest contributions to science. Certainly such trials have become increasingly important in assessing differences between competing treatments. The double-blind, placebo-controlled trial is now regarded as the 'gold standard' against which to judge all clinical trials. None the less many clinicians continue to harbour doubts about the ethics of such trials, and there remains much lively debate about how much information patients who are candidates for such trials should be given. Should they simply be made aware of the random allocation component of the trial, or should they be presented with the type of consent form suggested by Berry (1993), namely the following?:

I would like you to participate in a randomized clinical trial. We will in effect flip a coin and give you therapy A if a coin comes up heads and therapy B if it comes up tails. Neither you nor I will know which therapy you receive unless problems develop. (After presenting information about the therapies and their possible side effects:) No one really knows which therapy is better, and that is why we are conducting this trial. However we have had some experience with both therapies, including experience in the current trial. The available data suggest that you will live an average of five months longer on A than on B. But there is substantial variability in the data, and many people who have received B have lived longer than some patients on A. If I were you I would prefer A. My probability that you live longer on A is 25 per cent.

Your participation in this trial will help us treat other patients with this disease, so I ask in their name. But if you choose not to participate, you will receive whichever therapy you choose, including A or B.

It seems likely that the use of such an honest presentation would have the effect of severely limiting patient recruitment. So perhaps the 'informed consent' given by patients in many trials is not really so informed! The ethical issues involved in clinical trials are complex and involve philosophical and statistical arguments. But however complex, they do not, for most statisticians and for an increasing number of clinicians, outweigh the considerable advantages of properly conducted, randomized controlled trials.

FURTHER READING

Pocock, S. (1983). *Clinical trials: a practical approach.* Chichester and New York: John Wiley and Sons.

Guyatt, G.H., Sackett, D.L. and Cook, D.J. (1993). Users' guides to the medical literature. II. How to use an article about therapy or prevention A. Are the results of the study valid? *Journal of the American Medical Association* **270**, 2598–601.

Guyatt, G.H., Sackett, D.L. and Cook, D.J. (1993). Users' guides to the medical literature. II. How to use an article about therapy or prevention B. What were the results and will they help me in caring for my patients? *Journal of the American Medical Association* **271**, 59–63.

Inglefinger, J.A., Mosteller, F., Thibodeau, L.A. and Ware, J.H. (1983). *Biostatistics in Clinical Medicine.* New York: Macmillan. (Chapters 10 and 11.)

EXERCISES

1 The data given below were collected in a clinical trial of two treatments for anorexia nervosa in young women. The response variable used was the change in weight over a 12-week period. Patients were randomly allocated to the two treatments. Calculate the relevant confidence interval for assessing treatment difference (see Chapter 4).

Cognitive behavioural therapy		*Family therapy*	
Patient	Weight change (kg)*	Patient	Weight change (kg)*
1	2.3	1	12.0
2	0.7	2	11.0
3	−0.1	3	5.5
4	−0.7	4	9.4
5	−3.5	5	13.6
6	11.3	6	−2.9
7	3.5	7	−0.1
8	16.2	8	7.4
9	−6.5	9	21.5
10	1.6	10	−4.8
11	11.7	11	−5.3
12	6.1	12	13.4
13	1.1	13	13.0
14	−4.0	14	9.0
15	20.9	15	3.9
16	−9.1	16	5.7
17	2.1	17	10.7
18	−0.4	18	−1.1
19	1.4	19	1.0
20	−0.3	20	−3.0

*Negative values indicate a drop in weight.

2 Discuss possible advantages and disadvantages of a double-blind study. Can you give some examples where a double-blind study is clearly impossible? How could the virtues of 'blinding' be retained in such studies?

3 What arguments might you use to convince a clinician sceptical about the ethics of randomized controlled trials, that the alternatives are generally more objectionable?

4 Coronary artery disease involves a narrowing of the coronary
   arteries and often results in chest, neck and arm pains. Eventually the disease can lead to a myocardial infarction (heart
   attack) and possible death. Internal mammary artery ligation
   surgery is an operation designed to help with the problem and
   Battezzati *et al.* (1959) reported that amongst 304 cases who had
   the operation, 94.8% reported improvement. Clearly the operation was a great success. Or was it? Comment.

5 Two statisticians are asked by a clinician 'How large should my
   trial be?' The first undertakes some power calculations on the
   basis of information given by the clinician about possible effect,
   size etc. The second simply answers 'Use as many patients as you
   can afford and ethically justify!' Whose advice do you think the
   clinician should take and why?

Postscript:
Hypothesis Testing and
P-values

Statistical analysis of medical studies is based on the central idea that we make observations on a sample of subjects or patients and then draw inferences about the population from which the sample has been drawn. In general these inferences concern a population parameter or perhaps the difference between the corresponding parameters of two populations. The procedure used in this text for making such inferences has been by estimation and confidence intervals, the latter indicating the imprecision of sample statistics as estimates of population values.

But there is another approach to inference, that involving the *testing of hypotheses* through the use of *statistical significance tests*. Here the data are examined in relation to a statistical hypothesis about a population parameter and results given in terms of what is known as a **P-value**. Although we think the confidence interval method is to be preferred for reasons given later, it is important that the concept of a P-value is understood, since such values still appear frequently in the medical literature. So here is a very brief description in the form of a simple example.

TESTING WHETHER A POPULATION MEAN TAKES A PARTICULAR VALUE

Suppose we are interested in assessing whether or not the mean systolic blood pressure of a population of interest takes some particular value, say, $\mu = \mu_0$. Our sample mean has the value m. Now suppose that the distribution of blood pressures is Normal with a known standard deviation of σ. If this is the case, and if it is also true that the population mean is μ_0, then we know that on repeated sampling the sample mean, m, would be normally distributed with a mean μ_0 and standard error $\sigma/\text{sqrt}(N)$, where N is the sample size. Knowing this, it is now straightforward to ask 'How often will we observe a value of m for the sample mean, *or a value even further from* μ_0?' This probability, usually called the P-value, can be thought of as a measure of support for the hypothesis $\mu = \mu_0$: the lower its value the lower the support. Typically we decide that the support for the hypothesis is insufficient when the P-value drops below a particular threshold. This threshold is called the **significance level** of the test. If the observed P-value is equal to or lower than the significance level then we decide that there is sufficient evidence to reject the hypothesis $\mu = \mu_0$. If the P-value is above this value then we decide that we have insufficient evidence to reject the null hypothesis. The choice of what significance level to use is entirely arbitrary, the two most commonly used values being 0.05 (1/20) and 0.01 (1/100). To summarize, we start with a sample mean and a prior hypothesis about the value of the corresponding population mean and then ask 'What is the probability that we will get a sample mean this far from the population mean by chance?' If this probability is below say, 0.05, corresponding to a sample mean being 1.96 or more standard errors away from the postulated population mean, then we reject our hypothesis. We say that our result is **statistically significant** or that we have found a statistically significant departure from our initial hypothesis.

Very frequently we do not know the population's standard deviation σ and this also has to be estimated from our sample. Let the estimate be s. If we calculate the standard error of the mean using $s/\text{sqrt}(N)$, rather than $\sigma/\text{sqrt}(N)$, then the departure of the sample mean m from the population value μ divided by its standard error will not exactly follow the standard Normal distribution, but will follow a distribution characterized by having slightly larger tails. This distribution is called the **t-distribution**. The exact shape of a particular t-distribution will depend on its **degrees of freedom** which, in this case, are one less than the sample size (that is, $N-1$). As the degrees of freedom increase (that is, as the sample size increases) the corresponding t-distribution gets closer to the standard Normal distribution (the limiting case when N is infinitely large).

Now let us repeat the description of a significance test in a slightly more formal way. The construction of a significance test begins by setting up two hypotheses. The first, known as the **null hypothesis**, is that the population mean does take the value μ_0, and the other, the **alternative hypothesis**, that it does not take this value. The null hypothesis is frequently referred to as **H_0** and the alternative as **H_1**. To test the null hypothesis a sample of N observations is randomly drawn from the population of interest and is found to have a mean m and standard deviation s. Assuming that the population has a Normal distribution it can be shown that *if* the null hypothesis is true then the **test statistic**, t, given by

$$t = (m - \mu_0)/\text{s.e.}(m)$$

will be distributed following the t-distribution with $N-1$ degrees of freedom. Using tables of the t-distribution (that is, values of t with corresponding probabilities) we can determine the P-value associated with this test statistic. If the P-value is less than or equal to the predetermined significance level (often called **alpha**, or α) then we reject H_0 in favour of the alternative, H_1.

As a specific example, consider once again the quest to learn something about the average systolic blood pressure in a population of young men discussed in Chapter 4. Suppose a representative sample of 10 individuals from the population was found to have a mean of 130.0 mm Hg and a standard deviation of 10.6 mm Hg. We wish to use these data to assess the hypothesis that in the population the mean is 140 mm Hg. The test statistic calculated from the formula given above takes the value -2.98. The corresponding P-value is 0.015. The observed data give quite strong evidence against the null hypothesis. A value of t as extreme or more extreme than that observed would only be seen about once in a hundred times if the sample *did* arise from a population with a mean of 140. A 95% confidence interval for this example, constructed as described in previous chapters, would be (123.30, 136.70). As mentioned in Chapter 4, however, this confidence interval is approximate and applicable only to relatively large samples. Here the sample size is very small and the exact confidence interval might be more appropriate. This is obtained very easily by simply substituting the appropriate value from a t distribution with 9 degrees of freedom for the value 1.96 in the given formula provided in Chapter 4, the appropriate value being the one that 'cuts-off' 2.5% of the tails at either end of the distribution. From tables of the t distribution this is found to be the value 2.26, leading to the correct 95% confidence interval of (122.42, 137.58). The latter is a little wider than the one calculated earlier and this is generally true if the approximate method is used when the sample size is small.

There is an exact equivalence between the results of a significance test and those derived from the confidence interval approach, in the sense that all values within the 95% confidence interval for the population mean constructed from this sample, would, if used as the μ_0 value in H_0, give non-significant results. So in our example, all values in the interval (122.42, 137.58) if used for the null hypothesis value would lead to P-values greater than 0.05. Conversely all values outside this range would lead to declaring the results **significant at the 5% level**. Despite this equivalence, however, the confidence interval is far more useful in giving a range of values for the population mean, rather than assessing the significance or otherwise of one particular value.

The above was an example of the **t-test** for a single mean. A similar test can be constructed for assessing differences in population means. For dealing with proportions the relevant tests are the **chi-square** and **McNemar's test**. See Campbell and Machin (1993) for full details if required.

FURTHER READING

Gardner, M.J. and Altman, D.G. (1989). *Statistics with confidence.* London: British Medical Journal. (Chapter 2.)

Campbell, M.J. and Machin, D. (1993). *Medical statistics: a commonsense approach* (2nd edition). Chichester and New York: John Wiley and Sons.

Fischer, L.D. and van Belle, G. (1993). *Biostatistics: a methodology for the health sciences.* New York: John Wiley and Sons. (Chapter 4.)

References

Abramson, J.H. (1988). *Making sense of data: a self-instructional manual on the interpretation of epidemiological data*. Oxford: Oxford University Press.

Adelusi, B. (1977). Carcinoma of the cervix uteri in Ibadan: coital characteristics. *International Journal of Gynaecology and Obstetrics* **15**, 5–11.

Alderson, M. (1983). *An introduction to epidemiology* (2nd edition). London: Macmillan.

Armitage, P. and Berry, G. (1987). *Statistical methods in medical research* (2nd edition). Oxford: Blackwell Scientific.

Battezzati, M., Tagliaferro, A. and Cattanea, A.D. (1959). Clinical evaluation of bilateral internal mammary artery ligation as treatment of coronary heart disease. *American Journal of Cardiology* **4**, 180–3.

Baum, M.L., Arush, D.S., Chalmers, T.C., Sacks, H.S., Smith, H. and Fagerstrom, R.M. (1981). A survey of clinical trials of antibiotic prophylaxis in colon surgery: evidence against further use of no-treatment controls. *New England Journal of Medicine* **305**, 795–9.

Begg, C.B. and Berlin, J.A. (1988). Publication bias: a problem in interpreting medical data. *Journal of the Royal Statistical Society, Series A* **151**, 419–63.

Berry, D.A. (1993). A case for Bayesianism in clinical trials. *Statistics in Medicine* **12**, 1377–93.

Bland, M. (1987). *An introduction to medical statistics*. Oxford: Oxford University Press.

Bland, M. and Altman, D.G. (1986). Statistical methods for assessing agreement between two methods of clinical measurement. *Lancet* **i**, 307–10.

Bracken, M.B. (1987). Clinical trials and the acceptance of uncertainty. *British Medical Journal* **294**, 1111–12.

Breddin, K., Leoew, D., Lechner, K. and Uberla, E.W. (1979). Secondary prevention of myocardial infarction. Comparison of acetylsalicylic acid, phenprocoumon and placebo. A multi-center two-year prospective study. *Thrombosis and Hemostasis* **41**, 225–36.

Byar, D.P., Simon, R.M., Friedewald, W.T., Schlesselman, J.J., De Mets, D.L., Ellenberg, J.H., Gail, M.M. and Ware, J.H. (1976). Randomized clinical trials: perspectives on some recent ideas. *New England Journal of Medicine* **295**, 74–80.

Campbell, M.J. and Machin, D. (1993). *Medical statistics: a commonsense approach* (Second edition). Chichester and New York: John Wiley and Sons.

Chamberlain, G. (1991). Vital statistics of birth. *British Medical Journal* **303**, 178–81.

Clavel, F., Andrieu, N., Gairand, B., Bremond, A., Peana, L., Lansac, J., Breart, G., Rumeau-Rouquette, C., Flamant, R. and Renaud, R. (1991). Oral contraceptives and breast cancer: a French case-control study. *International Journal of Epidemiology* **20**, 32–8.

Cohen, J. (1960). A coefficient of agreement for nominal scales. *Educational and Psychological Measurement* **20**, 37–46.

Coulehan, J.L., Reisinger, K.S., Rogers, K.D. and Bradley, D.W. (1974). Vitamin C prophylaxis in a boarding school. *The New England Journal of Medicine*, **292**, 6–10

Doll, R. and Hill, A.B. (1954). The mortality of doctors in relation to their smoking habits. *British Medical Journal* **1**, 1451–5.

Doll, R. and Hill, A.B. (1964). Mortality in relation to smoking: ten years' observation of British doctors. *British Medical Journal* **1**, 1399–410 and 1460–7.

Dunn, G. (1989). *Design and analysis of reliability studies: statistical evaluation of measurement errors.* London: Edward Arnold.

Dunn, G. (1992). Design and analysis of reliability studies. *Statistical Methods in Medical Research* **1**, 123–57.

Elston, R.C. and Johnson, W.D. (1987). *Essentials of biostatistics.* Philadelphia: F. A. Davis Co.

Everitt, B.S. (1994). *Statistical methods for medical investigations* (Second edition). London: Edward Arnold.

Evidence-Based Medicine Working Group (1992). Evidence-based medicine. A new approach to teaching the practice of medicine. *Journal of the American Medical Association* **268**, 2420–5.

Fischer, L.D. and van Belle, G. (1993). *Biostatistics: a methodology for the health sciences.* New York: John Wiley and Sons.

Fischl, M.A. and the AZT collaborative working group (1987). The efficacy of azidothymidine (AZT) in the treatment of patients with AIDS and AIDS-related complex. *The New England Journal of Medicine* **317**, 185–97.

Fleiss, J.L. (1981). *Statistical methods for rates and proportions* (Second edition). New York: John Wiley and Sons.

Fleiss, J.L. (1987). Discussion contribution to Light, R.J. *Statistics in Medicine* **6**, 221–8.

Fleiss, J.L. (1993). The statistical basis of meta analysis. *Statistical Methods in Medical Research* **2**, 121–45.

Gardner, M.J. and Altman, D.G. (1989). *Statistics with confidence.* London: British Medical Journal.

Gehan, E.A. (1983). The evaluation of therapies: historical control studies. *Statistics in Medicine* **4**, 315–24.

Gehan, E.A. and Freireich, E.J. (1974). Non-randomized controls in cancer clinical trials. *New England Journal of Medicine* **290**, 198–203.

Goldberg, D.P. (1972). *The detection of psychiatric illness by questionnaire.* Maudsley Monograph No. 21. Oxford: Oxford University Press.

Gunnell, D.J. (1992). Mysterious slapped face rash at a holiday centre. *British Medical Journal* **304**, 477–9.

Guyatt, G.H., Sackett, D.L. and Cook, D.J. (1993). Users' guides to the medical literature. II. How to use an article about therapy or prevention B. Are the results of the study valid? *Journal of the American Medical Association* **270**, 2598–601.

Guyatt, G.H., Sackett, D.L. and Cook, D.J. (1993). Users' guides to the medical literature. II. How to use an article about therapy or prevention B. What were the results and will they help me in caring for my patients? *Journal of the American Medical Association* **271**, 59–63.

Hedlund, J.L. and Vieweg, B.W. (1979). The Hamilton Rating Scale for depression: a comprehensive review. *Journal of Operational Psychology* **10**, 149–65.

Heyting, A., Tolboom, J.T.B.M. and Essers, J.G.A. (1992). Statistical handling of dropouts in longitudinal clinical trials. *Statistics in Medicine* **11**, 2043–62.

Hill, A.B. (1962). *Statistical methods in clinical and preventive medicine.* Edinburgh: Livingstone.

Inglefinger, J.A., Mosteller, F., Thibodeau, L.A. and Ware, J.H.

(1983). *Biostatistics in Clinical Medicine*. New York: Macmillan.

Jaeschke, R., Guyatt, G. and Sackett, D.L. (1994). Users' guides to the medical literature. III. How to use an article about a diagnostic test A. Are the results of the study valid? *Journal of the American Medical Association* **271**, 389–91.

Jaeschke, R., Guyatt, G. and Sackett, D.L. (1994). Users' guides to the medical literature. III. How to use an article about a diagnostic test B. What are the results and will they help me in caring for my patients? *Journal of the American Medical Association* **271**, 703–7.

Janerich, D.T., Piper, J.M. and Glebatis, D.M. (1980). Oral contraceptives and birth defects. *American Journal of Epidemiology* **112**, 73–9.

Johnstone, E.C., Lawler, P. and Stevens, M. (1980). The Northwick Park electroconvulsive therapy trial. *Lancet* **ii**, 1317–20.

Landis, J.R. and Koch, G.C. (1977). The measurement of observer agreement for categorical data. *Biometrics* **33**, 159–74.

Lellouch, J. and Schwartz, D. (1971). L'essai thérapeutique: éthique individuelle ou éthique collective? *Rev. Inst. Int. Statist.* **39**, 127–36.

Lewis, T.L., Karlowski, T.R., Kapikian, A.Z., Lynch, J.M., Shaffer, G.W., Dennis, D.A. and Chalmers, T.C. (1975). A controlled clinical trial for ascorbic acid for the common cold. *Annals of New York Academy of Science* **258**, 505–12.

Lind, J. (1753). *A treatise of the scurvey*. Reprinted 1953. Edinburgh: Edinburgh University Press.

Maxwell, J.D., Patel, S.P., Bland, J.M., Lindsell, D.R.M. and Wilson, A.G. (1983). Chest radiography compared to laboratory markers in the detection of alcoholic liver disease. *Journal of the Royal College of Physicians* **17**, 220–3.

Meier, P. (1975). Statistics and medical experimentation. *Biometrics* **31**, 511–29.

Mitsuya, H., Weinhold, K.J. and Furman, P.A. (1985). 3′azido-3′-deoxythymidine: an antiviral agent that inhibits the infectivity and cytopathic effect of human T-lymphotropic virus type III/lymphadenopathy-associated virus *in vitro*. *Proceedings of the National Academy of Sciences, USA* **82**, 7096–100.

Newell, D.J. (1992). Intention-to-treat analysis: implications for quantitative and qualitative research. *International Journal of Epidemiology* **21**, 837–41.

Newman, H.H., Freeman, F.N. and Holzinger, K.J. (1937). *Twins.* Chicago: Chicago University Press.

Oakes, M. (1986). *Statistical inference: a commentary for the social and behavioural sciences.* Chichester and New York: John Wiley and Sons.

Oakes, M. (1993). The logic and role of meta-analysis in clinical research. *Statistical Methods in Medical Research* **2**, 147–60.

Oxman, A.D., Sackett, D.L. and Guyatt, G.H. (1993). Users' guides to the medical literature. I. How to get started. *Journal of the American Medical Association* **270**, 2093–5.

Patel, M., Gutzwiller, F., Paccaud, F. and Marazzi, A. (1989). A meta-analysis of acupuncture for chronic pain. *International Journal of Epidemiology* **18**, 900–6.

Pauling L., (1970). *Vitamin C and the common cold.* San Francisco: W. H. Freeman & Co.

Peduzzi, P., Detre, K., Wittes, J. and Holford, T. (1991). Intent-to-treat analysis and the problems of crossovers. An example from the Veterans Administration coronary bypass surgery study. *Journal of Thoracic and Cardiovascular Surgery* **101**, 481–7.

Peto, R. (1987). Discussion contribution to Light, R.J. *Statistics in Medicine* **6**, 221–8.

Pocock, S.J. (1983). *Clinical trials: a practical approach.* Chichester and New York: John Wiley and Sons.

Richman, D.D. and the AZT collaborative working group (1987). The toxicity of azidothymidine (AZT) in the treatment of patients with AIDS and AIDS-related complex. *New England Journal of Medicine* **317**, 192–7.

Sackett, D.L., Haynes, R.B., Guyatt, G.H. and Tugwell, P. (1991). *Clinical epidemiology* (Second Edition). Boston: Little, Brown.

Sacks, H.S., Chalmers, T.C. and Smith, H. (1983). Sensitivity and specificity of clinical trials: randomized vs historical controls. *Archives of Internal Medicine* **143**, 753–75.

Sartwell, P.E., Masi, A.T., Aerthes, F.G., Greene, G.R. and Smith, M.E. (1969). Thromboembolism and oral contraceptives: an epidemiological case-control study. *American Journal of Epidemiology* **90**, 365–75.

Shaw, L.W. and Chalmers, T. (1970). Ethics in co-operative clinical trials. *Annals of New York Academy of Science* **169**, 487–95.

Sivak, S.L. and Wormser, G.P. (1986). Predictive value of a screening test for antibodies to HTLV-III. *American Journal of Clinical Pathology* **85**, 700–3.

Smith, A.F. (1967). Diagnostic value of serum-creatine-kinase in a coronary-care unit. *Lancet* **ii**, 178–82.

Streiner, D.L. and Norman, G.R. (1989). *Health measurement scales. A practical guide to their development and use.* Oxford: Oxford University Press.

Strike, P. (1991). *Statistical methods in laboratory medicine.* Oxford: Butterworth.

Tufte, E.R. (1983). *The visual display of quantitative information.* Cheshire, CT, USA: Graphic Press.

United Kingdom National Case-Control Study Group (1989). Oral contraceptive use and breast cancer risk in young women. *Lancet* **i**, 973–82.

Yusuf, S., Peto, R., Lewis, J., Collins, R. and Sleight, P. (1985). Beta blockade during and after myocardial infarction. An overview of randomized trials. *Progress Cardiovascular Disease* **27**, 335–71.

Index